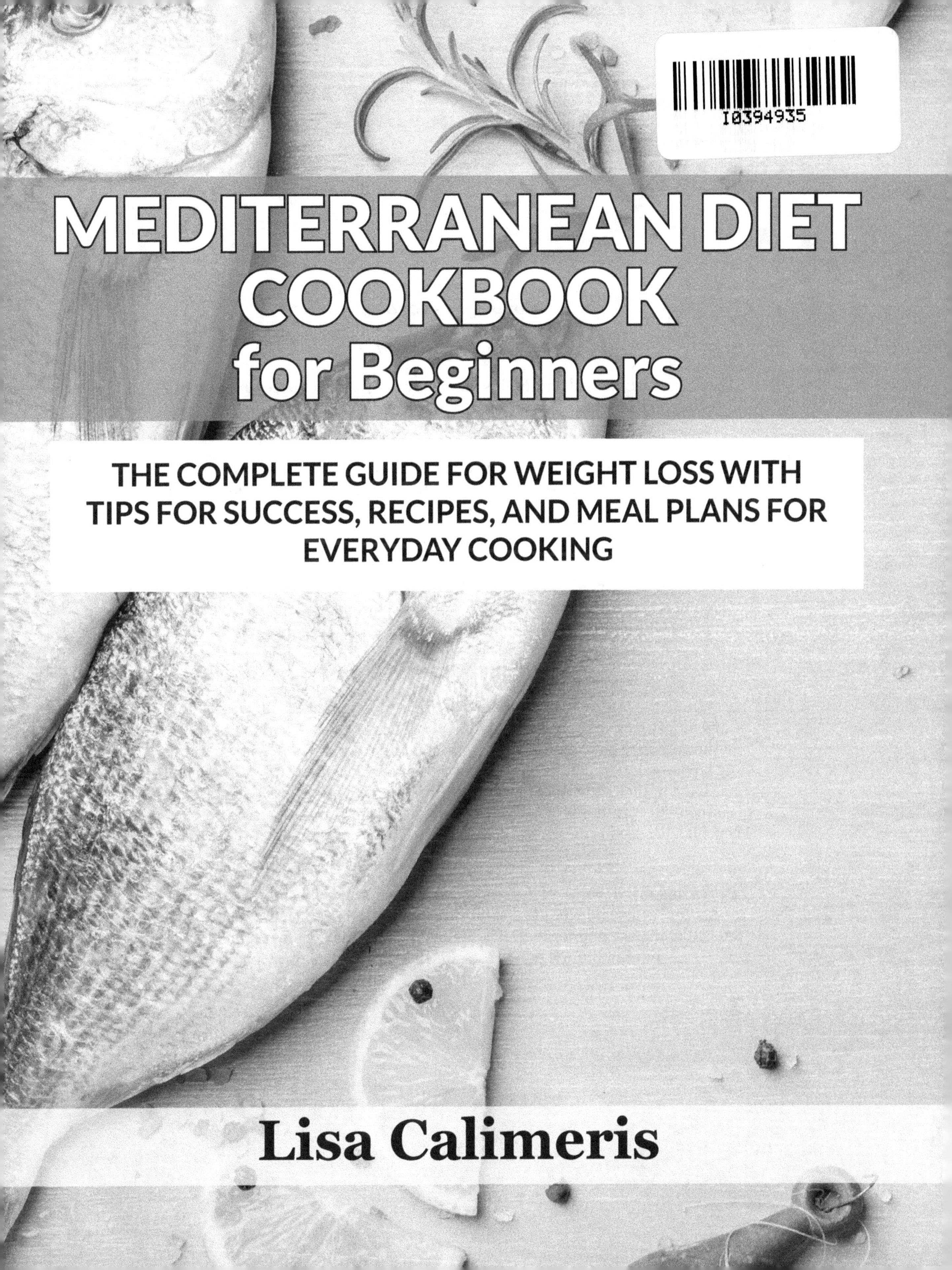

MEDITERRANEAN DIET COOKBOOK for Beginners

THE COMPLETE GUIDE FOR WEIGHT LOSS WITH TIPS FOR SUCCESS, RECIPES, AND MEAL PLANS FOR EVERYDAY COOKING

Lisa Calimeris

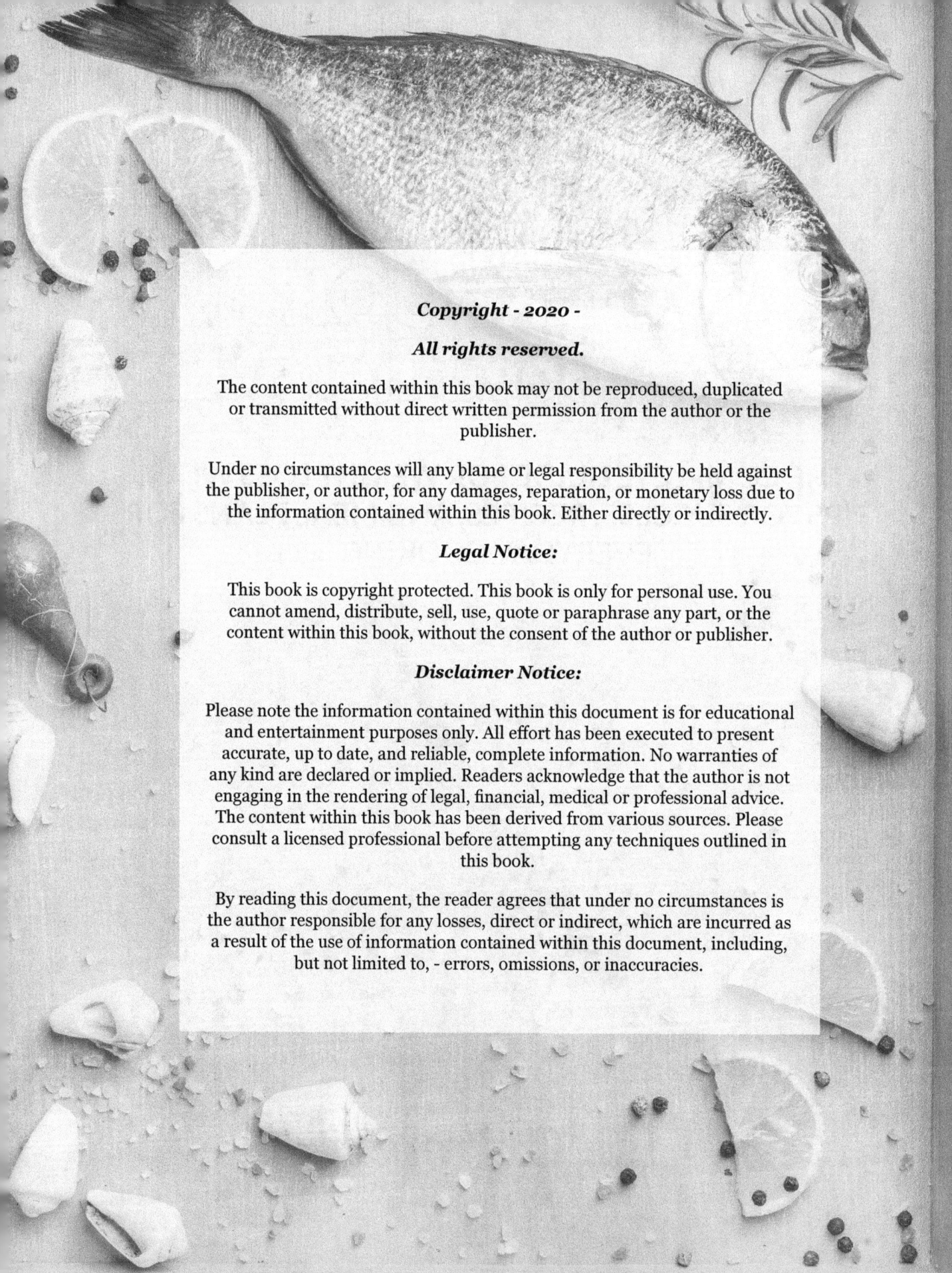

Copyright - 2020 -

All rights reserved.

The content contained within this book may not be reproduced, duplicated or transmitted without direct written permission from the author or the publisher.

Under no circumstances will any blame or legal responsibility be held against the publisher, or author, for any damages, reparation, or monetary loss due to the information contained within this book. Either directly or indirectly.

Legal Notice:

This book is copyright protected. This book is only for personal use. You cannot amend, distribute, sell, use, quote or paraphrase any part, or the content within this book, without the consent of the author or publisher.

Disclaimer Notice:

Please note the information contained within this document is for educational and entertainment purposes only. All effort has been executed to present accurate, up to date, and reliable, complete information. No warranties of any kind are declared or implied. Readers acknowledge that the author is not engaging in the rendering of legal, financial, medical or professional advice. The content within this book has been derived from various sources. Please consult a licensed professional before attempting any techniques outlined in this book.

By reading this document, the reader agrees that under no circumstances is the author responsible for any losses, direct or indirect, which are incurred as a result of the use of information contained within this document, including, but not limited to, - errors, omissions, or inaccuracies.

Table of Contents

CHAPTER 1:
INTRODUCTION — 8

CHAPTER 2:
UNDERSTANDING THE MEDITERRANEAN DIET — 10

CHAPTER 3:
THE HEALTH BENEFITS OF THE MEDITERRANEAN DIET — 16

CHAPTER 4:
WHY THE MEDITERRANEAN DIET? — 20

CHAPTER 5:
STARTING THE MEDITERRANEAN DIET — 24

CHAPTER 6:
MEDITERRANEAN DIET FOOD PYRAMID — 26

CHAPTER 7:
SMOOTHIE RECIPES — 28

1. SWEET KALE SMOOTHIE — 29
2. CRANBERRY-PUMPKIN SMOOTHIE — 30
3. CHOCOLATE BANANA SMOOTHIE — 31
4.. FRUIT SMOOTHIE — 32
5. MANGO-PEAR SMOOTHIE — 33
6. AVOCADO-BLUEBERRY SMOOTHIE — 34
7. BLUEBERRY BANANA PROTEIN SMOOTHIE — 35
8. HONEY AND WILD BLUEBERRY SMOOTHIE — 36
9. OATS BERRY SMOOTHIE — 37
10. HEARTY PEAR AND MANGO SMOOTHIE — 38
11. FIG SMOOTHIE WITH CINNAMON — 39
12. RASPBERRY VANILLA SMOOTHIE — 40
13. KALE-PINEAPPLE SMOOTHIE — 41

CHAPTER 8: BREAKFAST RECIPES 42

14. GREEK BOWL 43
15. MORNING OATS 44
16. YOGURT WITH DATES 45
17. SPINACH FRITTATA 46
18. BAKED EGGS WITH PARSLEY 47
19. MUSHROOM CASSEROLE 48
20. VANILLA PANCAKES 49
21. SAVORY EGG GALETTES 50
22. ARUGULA FRITTATA 51
23. BREAKFAST TOAST 52
24. ARTICHOKE OMELET 53
25. BELL PEPPER FRITTATA 54

CHAPTER 9: SALADS AND SOUPS 56

26. TOMATO, CUCUMBER, AND FETA SALAD 57
27. GOAT CHEESE STUFFED TOMATOES 58
28. CLASSIC TABBOULEH 59
29. MEDITERRANEAN GREENS 60
30. NORTH AFRICAN ZUCCHINI SALAD 61
31. AVOCADO SALAD 62
32. TUNISIAN STYLE CARROT SALAD 63
33. CLASSIC GREEK SALAD 64
34. CHICKEN LEEK SOUP 65
35. MEATBALL SOUP 66
36. LEMON LAMB SOUP 67
37. EGGPLANT SOUP 68

CHAPTER 10: PASTA, RICE, AND COUSCOUS 70

38. BREAKFAST COUSCOUS 71
39. PORK WITH COUSCOUS 72
40. TUNA AND COUSCOUS 73
41. GARLIC RICE 74

42. CARROT RICE	75
43. SEAFOOD AND VEGGIE PASTA	76
44. ALETHEA'S LEMONY ASPARAGUS PASTA	77
45. MUSHROOM AND VEGETABLE PENNE PASTA	78
46. BROCCOLI AND ORECCHIETTE PASTA WITH FETA	79
47. FIBER PACKED CHICKEN RICE	80
48. TASTY GREEK RICE	81

CHAPTER 11: SEAFOOD AND FISH RECIPES — 82

49. GRILLED FISH ON LEMONS	83
50. VINEGAR HONEYED SALMON	84
51. ORANGE FISH MEAL	85
52. SHRIMP ZOODLES	86
53. TUNA NUTTY SALAD	87
54. SALMON SKILLET SUPPER	88
55. WEEKNIGHT SHEET PAN FISH DINNER	89
56. CRISPY POLENTA FISH STICKS	90
57. TUSCAN TUNA AND ZUCCHINI BURGERS	91
58. ASPARAGUS TROUT MEAL	92
59. KALE OLIVE TUNA	93
60. TANGY ROSEMARY SHRIMPS	94
61. ASPARAGUS SALMON	95
62. SICILIAN KALE AND TUNA BOWL	96
63. MEDITERRANEAN COD STEW	97

CHAPTER 12: POULTRY RECIPES — 98

64. CACCIATORE BLACK OLIVE CHICKEN	99
65. MUSTARD GREEN CHICKEN	100
66. CHICKPEA SPICED CHICKEN	101
67. VEGETABLE RICE CHICKEN	102
68. TENDER CHICKEN QUESADILLA	103
69. LIGHT CAESAR	104
70. CHICKEN PARM	105
71. CHICKEN BOLOGNESE	106

72. CHICKEN SHAWARMA   107
73. CAPRESE CHICKEN DINNER   108

CHAPTER 13:
MEAT AND EGGS RECIPES   110

74. MEDITERRANEAN GRILLED PORK CHOPS   111
75. SIMPLE PORK STIR FRY   112
76. PORK AND LENTIL SOUP   113
77. SIMPLE BRAISED PORK   114
74. MEDITERRANEAN GRILLED PORK CHOPS   115
78. CAPRESE POACHED EGGS   116
79. SAUTÉED GREENS AND EGGS   117
80. SLOW-COOKED MEDITERRANEAN PORK   118
81. PORK AND BEAN STEW   119
82. GLUTEN-FREE PORTOBELLO PESTO EGG OMELET   120
83. FETA BAKED EGGS   121
84. EASY ROASTED PORK SHOULDER   122
85. HERB ROASTED PORK   123
86. SLOW COOKED BEEF BRISKET   124
87. MEDITERRANEAN BEEF DISH   125
88. BEEF TARTARE   126
89. MEATBALLS AND SAUCE   127
90. POACHED EGGS   128

CHAPTER 14:
VEGETARIAN RECIPES   130

91. ROASTED VEGETABLES AND CHICKPEAS   131
92. VEGGIE RICE BOWLS WITH PESTO SAUCE   132
93. SAUTÉED SPINACH AND LEEKS   133
94. VEGAN SESAME TOFU AND EGGPLANTS   134
95. VEGETARIAN COCONUT CURRY   135
96. ZOODLES WITH BEET PESTO   136
97. SWEET POTATO CHICKPEA BUDDHA BOWL   137
98. EASY ZUCCHINI PATTIES   138
99. ZUCCHINI CRISP   139

CHAPTER 15: SANDWICHES AND WRAPS — 140

- 100. MEDITERRANEAN EGG WHITE BREAKFAST SANDWICH — 141
- 101. MEDITERRANEAN LETTUCE WRAPS — 142
- 102. SHRIMP, AVOCADO, AND FETA WRAP — 143
- 103. FLATBREAD SANDWICHES — 144
- 104. BEAN LETTUCE WRAPS — 145
- 105. ITALIAN TUNA SANDWICHES — 146
- 106. DILL SALMON SALAD WRAPS — 147

CHAPTER 16: DESSERTS AND FRUITS — 148

- 107. MASCARPONE AND FIG CROSTINI — 149
- 108. CRUNCHY SESAME COOKIES — 150
- 109. ALMOND COOKIES — 151
- 110. BAKLAVA AND HONEY — 152
- 111. DATE AND NUT BALLS — 153
- 112. MANGO SNOW — 154
- 113. MINTY COCONUT CREAM — 155
- 114. WATERMELON CREAM — 156
- 115. GRAPES STEW — 157
- 116. COCOA SWEET CHERRY CREAM — 158
- 117. CREAMY RICE PUDDING — 159
- 118. RICOTTA-LEMON CHEESECAKE — 160
- 119. CROCKPOT KETO CHOCOLATE CAKE — 161
- 120. KETO CROCKPOT CHOCOLATE LAVA CAKE — 162

CHAPTER 17: TIPS ON HOW TO LIVE THE MEDITERRANEAN DIET LIFESTYLE — 163

CHAPTER 18: 2-WEEK MEAL PLAN — 166

CONCLUSION — 168

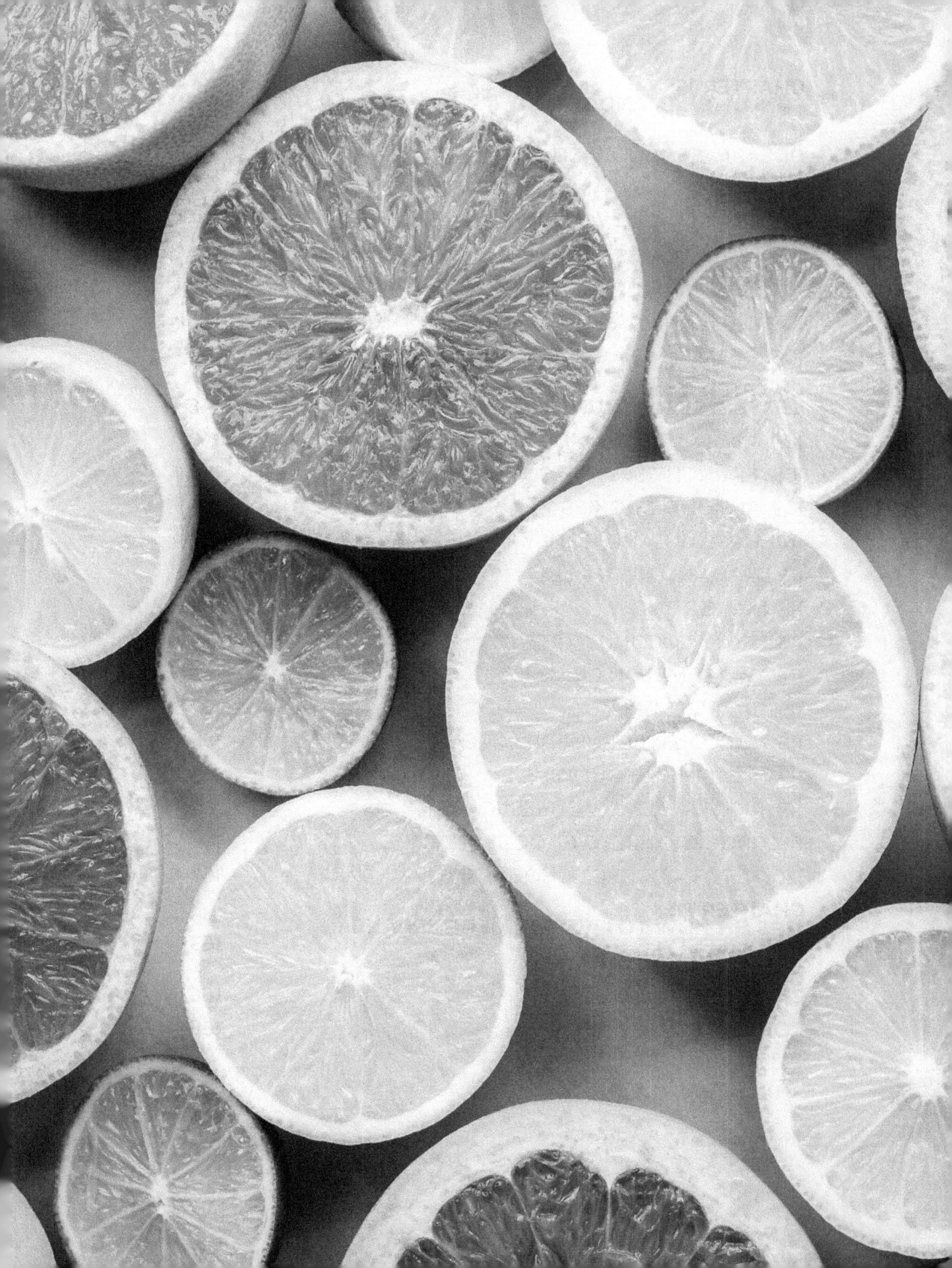

CHAPTER 1:
Introduction

You may be wondering what exactly the Mediterranean diet is, and you need to be aware that it's more of a lifestyle than a normal diet. It's a way of eating that will help you to live a full and happy life. You can lose weight and strengthen your heart while providing yourself with all of the nutrients you need for a long, healthy life. Those that follow this diet are often at a lower risk of cancer and Alzheimer's disease, enjoy an extended lifespan, and overall have better cardiovascular health. The Mediterranean diet consists of foods that are rich in healthy oils, filled with vegetables and fruit, and foods that are low in saturated fat.

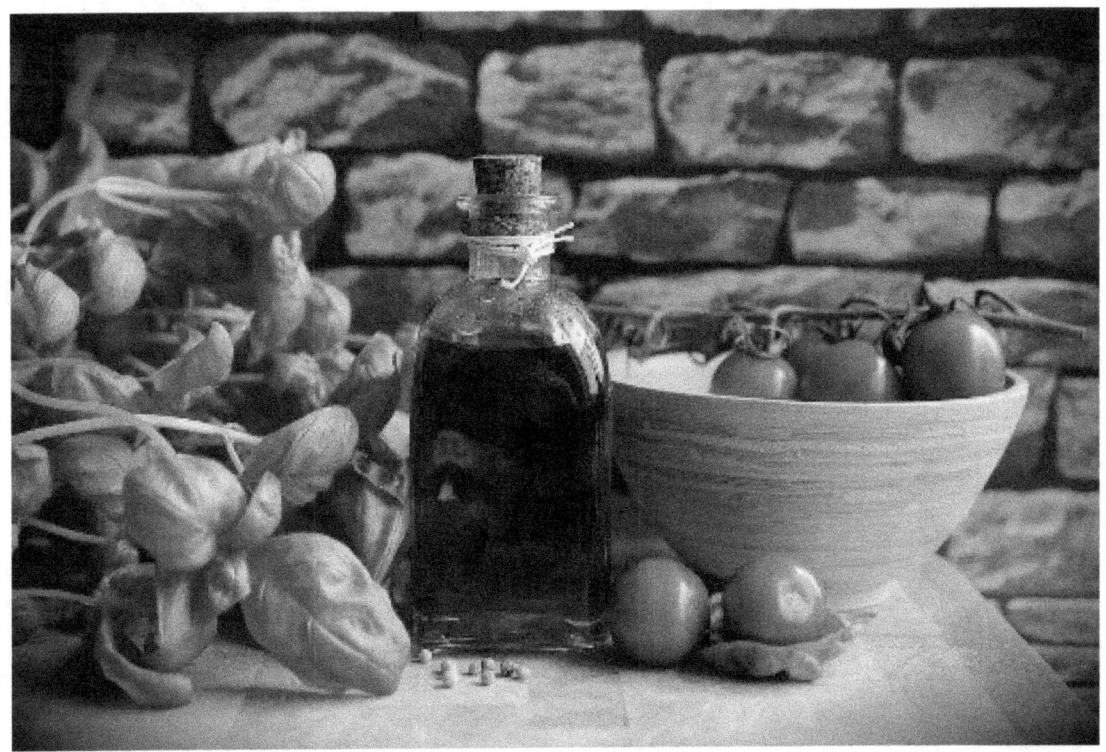

This is a heart-healthy eating plan that's based on the food that can be found in the Mediterranean, which includes quite a number of countries. It includes pasta, rice, vegetables, and fruit, but it does not allow for much red meat. Nuts are also a part of this diet, but they should be limited due to the fact that they are high in fat and calories.

The Mediterranean diet limits your fat consumption and discourages the eating of saturated or trans-fats. Both types have been linked to heart disease. Grains are often served whole and bread is an important part of the lifestyle, but butter doesn't really play a role. Wine, however, has a huge place in the Mediterranean diet both in cooking and including a glass with each meal if you are of age. The primary sources of fat in this diet are olive oil and fatty fish including herring, mackerel, albacore, tuna, sardines, salmon, and trout, which are rich in omega-3 fatty acids.

With the Mediterranean diet, you are giving your body the nutrients and vitamins it needs, so you won't feel hungry. However, it requires a large commitment to eating natural foods, removing temptation, and cooking regular meals. If you love to cook this isn't much of a change, but for those that have few skills in the kitchen it can be a daunting, but well rewarding task. Of course, like with any diet stay,good hydration and moderate exercise will go a long way!

CHAPTER 2:
Understanding the Mediterranean Diet

The Mediterranean diet is inspired by the eating habits of the populations around the Mediterranean Sea. The populations of southern Italy and Greece are the main regions that influence this diet. But it isn't the diet that is consumed today in many of these regions that gained so much attention. The Mediterranean diet refers to the traditional eating habits and lifestyles of these areas in the 1950s and 1960s. It was during this time that researchers noticed a significant difference in the health of populations in these areas when compared to those living in America. It was obvious that many of the individuals in the Mediterranean areas were healthier and the key difference between those living in the Mediterranean and those living in America was their diet.

If you decide to follow the Mediterranean diet, the establishment of your diet will be natural products, vegetables, whole-grain bread, pasta, rice, grains, and potatoes, alongside beans, nuts, vegetables, and seeds. These foods ought to be consumed day by day and will shape the premise of each meal you eat, with crisp vegetables becoming the overwhelming focus. While carbohydrates are a piece of this diet, they will, in general, be entire, unpredictable, high in fiber, and consumed with protein or fats simultaneously.

Fish and seafood are the staple proteins in this diet. Ordinary consumption of oily fish, similar to salmon, mackerel, and fish, assists with satiety and also lifts admission of heart solid omega-3 unsaturated fats. When looking for fish, be that as it may, avoid ranch-raised fish at whatever point conceivable. Extra wellsprings of fat incorporate olive and canola oil, which replace margarine and grease for cooking and dressing food.

With some restraint, you'll eat poultry, eggs, cheddar, and plain, unsweetened yogurt every other day or a couple of times each week relying upon your inclination. Decide on characteristic dairy and cheddar, not vigorously handled or seasoned assortments, to avoid added additives, sugars, or synthetics. Goat cheddar and feta cheddar are normally observed on Mediterranean diet menus.

Desserts such as crude nectar are appreciated in exacting control, while different treats are eaten distinctly on extraordinary events. Red meat is barely consumed in the Mediterranean diet, alongside exceptionally handled meats like wieners and bacon. In addition, a solitary glass of wine is considered a staple in the diet and part of what makes the diet so heart solid, so don't feel bad about presenting yourself with a glass with your supper.

WHO IS THIS DIET WELL SUITED FOR?

This diet will work well for someone who wants to boost the well-being of their heart, reduce their cholesterol, lose some weight, and do without feeling insulted as such. Note, though, if you consume too many processed grains in your diet (white bread, white pasta, and so on), this will potentially build up your cholesterol level, so it's important to concentrate on healthier grains that have been handled as poorly as you would expect under the circumstances.

This diet is likewise extraordinary for the individuals who don't react well to a conventional low carb diet. A significant piece of the Mediterranean diet is the worth set on regular exercise, which is bolstered by the vitality you'll get from complex carbohydrates and common natural product sugars. Try not to be amazed if 50-60% of your all-out everyday calorie consumption originates from carbohydrates while on this plan.

At last, the plan is extraordinary for the individuals who are hoping to keep up their weight utilizing a dietary convention that can be supported for quite a long time to come. Since you are not dispensing with any food groups altogether, it's truly conceivable to get balanced nutrition with this plan.

BASIC GUIDING PRINCIPLES
CONSUME LOTS OF FRUIT

There isn't any limit in regard to the selection of fruit to include on the MD. However, since culmination includes nutrients in special quantities, it is always higher to go along with a darkish-colored end result, which nutritionists claim to supply a morenormal dietary punch. Dark-colored fruits, particularly the darkish crimson and orange ones, and even veggies provide antioxidants and phytonutrients. Variety is likewise a vital aspect in choosing fruits for the MD.

The following fruits are usually grown within the Mediterranean: figs, grapes, lemons, mandarin oranges, olives, persimmons, and pomegranates. Other important culminationson the MD are blackberries, blueberries, cranberries, plums, red grapes, and crimson raspberries. MD experts also recommend succulent fruit or those containing lots of fiber and water, such as apples, oranges, peaches, and watermelons. The idea behind more water and fiber in the diet is to help weight watchers experience gladness longer and to aid in the digestive process.

CONSUME LOTS OF VEGETABLES

All vegetables can be included in the MD; however, people need to attempt to restrict their intake of corn and white potatoes because of their high starch content, which in turn contributes to extra calories. The following greens are commonly grown inside the Mediterranean: artichokes, asparagus, broccoli, broccoli rabe, cabbage, eggplant, green beans, garlic, onions, and tomatoes. Dark-colored vegetables along with beets, carrots, purple peppers, and sweet potatoes are super sources of antioxidants and phytonutrients. Likewise, eat masses of fresh, leafy veggies aside from broccoli due to the fact these also are powerhouses of nutrients: bok choy, cauliflower, collards, kale, lettuce, mustard, romaine, spinach, summertime and wintry weather squash, turnip vegetables, and zucchini.

Adults need to consume several cups of veggies on the MD. Vegetables can be eaten raw, cooked, or used as elements in different dishes. Those who would love to strive for the MD but are nevertheless hesitating due to the fact they don't want to eat loads of vegetables might be glad to recognize that vegetable serving sizes do now not need to be large. The following common vegetable consumption requirements can also serve as your manual in getting ready food the Mediterranean way. The good news is that it conforms to the dietary pointers of health and nutrition authorities:

At least 1 ½ cups of orange-colored greens in keeping with the week. At least 2 cups according to week of darkish inexperienced greens.

At least 5 ½ cups in line with a week of other vegetables.

For the ones trying the MD for healthy eating, at least 2 ½ cups in keeping with a week of starchy veggies, however, the ones doing the MD for weight loss must refrain from or limit intake of starch-rich veggies to a maximum of one cup in a week.

CONSUME LEGUMES
Legumes are complete within the macronutrients carbohydrates, proteins, fats, and oils, whereas the end result and vegetables do not now have fat and oils. Legumes are also wealthy in vitamins B1, B3, B6, and B9 and in minerals inclusive of calcium, magnesium, and molybdenum. The following legumes are usually grown within the Mediterranean: chickpeas, lentils, and peas. However, legumes for inclusion within the MD are infinite and may also encompass black beans, black-eyed peas, great northern beans, kidney beans, and cut up beans.

INCLUDE NUTS AND SEEDS IN YOUR DIET
Nuts and seeds are a staple in Mediterranean cuisine, both as the principal element in a snack recipe or to add fantastic flavor to food. The following nuts are typically grown in the Mediterranean: almonds, hazelnuts, pine nuts, and walnuts. Other healthy nuts and seeds which are indispensable in the MD are: Brazil nuts, cashew nuts, chia seeds, flaxseeds or linseeds, macadamia nuts, peanuts (even though peanuts are actually legumes), pecan nuts, pistachio nuts, pumpkin seeds, sesame seeds, and sunflower seeds. Quinoa (absolutely now not a true cereal but a pseudocereal) may be considereda seed.

With all the remarkable advantages which may be derived from nuts and seeds (especially healthy fats), those food items also incorporate calories. Those who are looking at their weight or are following the MD weight-reduction plan for weight loss need to control their intake of nuts and seeds.

Here are approximate numbers of a few nuts that normally include an ounce - the everyday serving size of nuts:

- Almonds: 20 to 25
- Brazil nuts: 6 to 8
- Cashew nuts: 16 to 18
- Hazelnuts: 10 to 12
- Peanuts: 28
- Pecan nuts: 15 halves
- Pine nuts: 50 to 157
- Pistachios: 45 to 47
- Walnuts: 14 halves

A caveat about nuts: Brazil nuts, cashew nuts, and peanuts have higher content material of unhealthy fats. The high-quality nuts are almonds and walnuts because of their Omega-3 content and their splendid taste. Nuts are satisfactory when they're raw, but if you really need to cook them then go for toasted nuts. Also, ensure that they may be unsalted and uncoated, and with no added sugar or fat. Also, the claims about chia seeds have not but been scientifically proven, so they should be eaten up in mild servings of one ounce at the most

Eat entire grains, in particular whole-grain bread.Technically, the term whole-grain refers back to the grain or method grain products wherein the caryopsis such as the anatomical components bran, germ, and endosperm are intact whether they're ground, cracked, or flaked. Whole grains are necessary to the MD as they contain excessive quantities of fiber and impart natural goodness to food. Among the entire grain produce commonplace within the Mediterranean region are barley, corn, rice, and wheat. If you like bread, then select dense, heavy, chewy bread baked from white wheat, barley, and oats. If you love pasta, pick out whole-grain pasta products from the grocery store.

There are many motives for deciding on whole-grain foods. This includes not only health benefits but additionally for that feeling of fullness you want for your everyday routines. MD experts additionally endorse steel-cut, entire-grain oatmeal, and multi-grain hot cereals. The good information with MD is that it allows for a wide preference for whole grains. Even people who love rice can enjoy ingesting rice so long as they choose brown rice. Couscous and polenta are also amazing entire grain choices.

Whole grains are a fundamental part of the Mediterranean weight-reduction plan.

USE OLIVE OIL IN COOKING AND IN SALADS

Olive oil is the main fat supply used within the MD. Thus, the consumption of olive oil in Mediterranean countries is excessive even as other less expensive oils are becoming famous. With the cutting-edge interest in MD, even non-Mediterranean international locations together with Germany, Japan, UK, and the US have increasing consumption of olive oil. Olive oil defines the distinctive taste of the MD and is therefore of precise significance within the overall context of the MD.

Olive oil is not only effective for increasing the palatability of foods, but also improves the feel and complements the taste. In Greece, the very famous lathera dish consists of veggies cooked in an olive oil-based total sauce, tomatoes, and garlic. Leading authorities on the MD believe that without the use of olive oil within the instruction of Mediterranean dishes, it might be practically impossible for humans in Greece and inside the surrounding international locations inside the area to consume high quantities of greens and legumes.

Olive oil is used inside the Mediterranean weight-reduction plan and in addition is also used for the following functions among others:

- Raw olive oil is used in aioli and other dips.
- Vegetable marinades.
- Flavoring for soups and stews by using long, slow cooking, especially in pistou and for batter, dough, and numerous pastries.
- Bread with oil, which is taken into consideration as elemental Mediterranean cuisine, which includes the Catalan dish pa amb oli.

Mediterranean people veryrarely use butter in their cuisine, and they no longer omit it because olive oil has its simple appeal for his or her dishes. In activities in which olive oil does no longer suit a particular recipe, canola oil is used instead. Extra virgin olive oil, mainly the lighter model, is the best preference for salad dressings, for use in meals eaten raw, and in baking. However, for cooking, everyday extra virgin oil found in the supermarket is just fine. One should no longer hesitate to put together foods the Mediterranean way due to the price of olive oil because it will replace butter and margarine. The small fee delivered in the use of olive is nothing compared to its health advantages.

INCLUDE MODERATE AMOUNTS OF LOW-FAT DAIRY OR IF POSSIBLE, NON-FAT DAIRY

In the Mediterranean, goat and sheep milk are more desired than cow's milk. However, as long as you select low-fat or non-fat milk, it's miles more sufficient for inclusion within the MD. Rather than the standard Western cheese, yogurt is a very crucial constituent of the MD, collectively with some hard and soft forms of cheese. Greek yogurt has a rich silky texture and is widely available in many supermarkets in the US. It is preferable because it has two times the protein content of regular commercial yogurt but costs the same as the ordinary name-brand yogurt.

There is even fat-unfastened Greek yogurt for weightwatchers which is already available within the US. Even Starbucks has jumped into the Greek yogurt bandwagon and is teaming up with a Greek yogurt manufacturer. By next year, Americans established with the healthful Mediterranean weight loss program can buy ready-to-consume Greek yogurt parfaits from the multi-chain international espresso store.

Meanwhile, the MD isn't always acknowledged for its heavy use of cheese. Rather, cheese is used extra as a flavoring to decorate the taste of food, not necessary to overwhelm it. Cheese is also utilized in MD in combination with dessert. If you want cheese, make sure that it is also the low-fat variety and consume dairy products in moderation.

EAT FISH AND SHELLFISH
Influenced by way of geography, the Mediterranean weight loss program includes seafood as one of its crucial components. Moreover, the selection of fish in the traditional eating regimen is largely responsible for the coronary heart-healthy popularity of the MD weight loss program. Fish like cod, haddock, mackerel, red mullet, salmon, and sardines, which can be cold-water fish varieties, are rich in Omega-3 and different unsaturated fats. Squid and octopus also are staple seafood in the MD. Consuming fish with high Omega-3 rather than animal meats guarantees that the body's arteries are not clogged and are protected from coronary diseases.

Other fish now not essential from the Mediterranean which might be rich in Omega-3 and unsaturated fats are albacore, tuna, anchovies, Arctic char or iwana, Atlantic mackerel, sablefish or black cod, Pacific halibut, rainbow trout, shad, smelt, and wild salmon. Shellfish are also welcome in the MD. Among the healthiest are clams, crab, lobster, mussels, oysters, scallops, and shrimps.

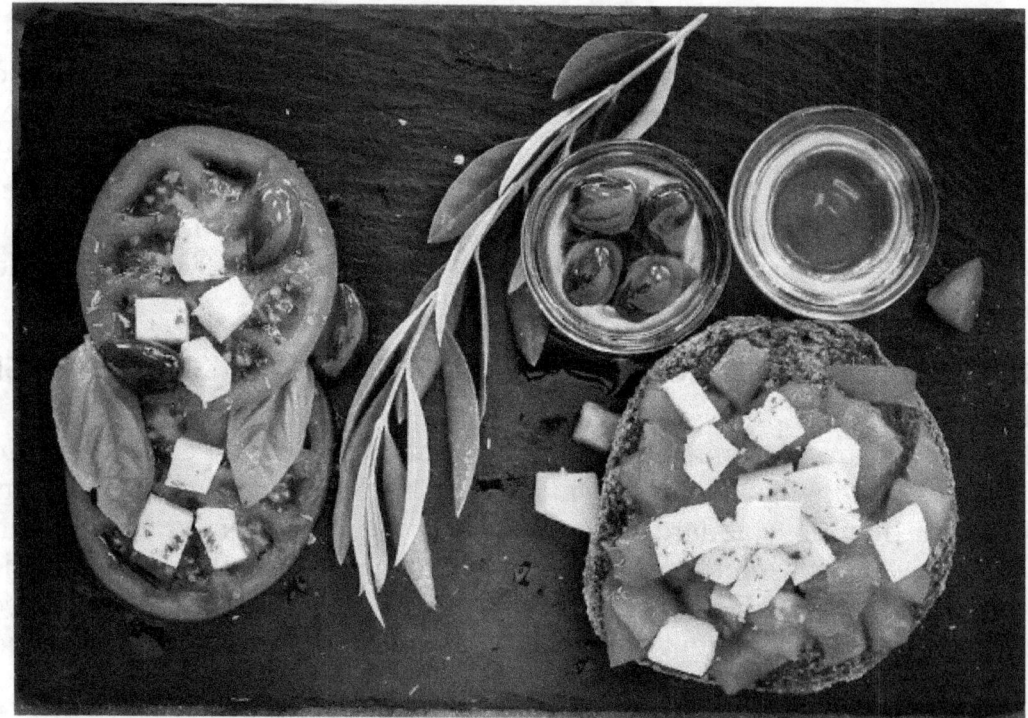

CHAPTER 3:
The Health Benefits of the Mediterranean Diet

The Mediterranean lifestyle's health benefits have become so successful for so many people. It has more benefits than just losing some extra weight! You can improve many health conditions like type-2 diabetes or heart disease, and even help improve other facets of your health like acne, mental acuity, and hopefully extend the overall longevity of your lifespan. These aren't just people's experiences with the diet, but scientific research that has been conducted to find what the diet's benefits are.

What are some of the astounding health benefits possible on the Mediterranean diet? Here are some possibilities of how you could improve your health:

Losing weight and keeping it off! To many people, one of the best and most appealing benefits of the Mediterranean diet is that you are able to lose weight by making healthier eating decisions. You do not have to starve yourself or cut your food portions, but by naturally shifting to more healthier foods, you can lose weight and keep that weight off. It's all about which foods you are eating to gain your nutrients. For example, you're staying away from red meat and relying on things like fish, legumes, and seafood as your sources of protein. You're also eating fresh fruits and vegetables which are packed with essential vitamins, minerals, and fiber that keep you full in between meals. You've also cut out the unhealthy items from your diet like sugar, processed foods, and refined bread. Some people may just start the Mediterranean diet to lose weight, so this may be the first goal they reach before they learn they can achieve many others!

Keeps your heart healthy and reduces risk factors of cardiovascular heart disease. As we mentioned in the previous chapter, there are many factors of the Mediterranean diet that improve heart health such as the addition of olive oil and wine. Olive oil is high in alpha-linolenic acid (ALA) which has been found to decrease the risk of cardiac or premature death by almost 30%. Compared to other oils like sunflower oil or vegetable oil, only olive oil has been found to significantly lower blood pressure. With a healthier diet focused on good fats, the Mediterranean diet can also maintain the HDL cholesterol in the body, the "good" cholesterol, and decrease the LDL "bad" cholesterol. Not only that, but it also reduces the level of unhealthy fatty triglycerides in the blood. A high level of these has been linked to an increased risk of stroke or sudden cardiac death. With the improvement of these risk factors, the body can have better blood flow and fewer plaque build-ups which keeps the arteries open and blood steadily pumping throughout the body. A study found that when obese men followed the Mediterranean diet, they had better blood flow compared to when they ate junk food, and their arteries did not dilate.

Improves the longevity of your life. We have no guarantee of our future, but research shows that the Mediterranean lifestyle may have the ability to increase your lifespan. A famous study called the Lyon Diet Heart Study followed patients who had suffered from heart attacks between 1988 and 1992. They were told to follow either a normal post-heart attack low-fat diet recommended by doctors at the time or the Mediterranean diet. Nearly 4 years after the study started, researchers found that the group who followed the Mediterranean diet had nearly 70% less risk of heart disease and 50% less risk of death than the followers of the low-fat diet. This longevity was also very much visible in the people of the Mediterranean that Ancel Keys first studied when he found the link between diet and quality of life. With all the benefits of the Mediterranean diet in improving your health, such as reducing the risk of cancer, heart disease, and neurodegenerative diseases, it's only logical that this will keep you healthy for longer. All by simply changing the types of food you're eating! Fresh fruits and vegetables tend to contain higher antioxidants which are great for strengthening your immune system and preventing disease.

Maintains eye vision and health. The Mediterranean diet includes a high amount of fish which means a high intake of omega 3 fatty acids. Unlike other triglycerides, these molecules play an important role in eye health. The American Academy of Ophthalmology ranks the Mediterranean diet as one of the best diets to protect and maintain eye health. Combined with the frequent servings of fish and seafood a week, there are also fresh fruits and vegetables that contain antioxidants. Studies show that having fish just once a week can decrease your chances of eye damage that can commonly occur in people over the age of 50, such as cataracts or cloudy vision. With the Mediterranean diet, you're having fish many times a week! Most of the general public doesn't have enough fish so they supplement with fish oil tablets, but with the Mediterranean diet, you'll be getting more than enough fatty acids. Fatty acids are also present in nuts and seeds which are a recommended snack in between meals.

Improves mental focus and cognitive functioning. Omega-3 fatty acids are composed of two parts: DHA and EPA. Along with vision health, as we mentioned above, they are also vital in brain development and functioning. They help preserve the health of brain cells and improve the communication between brain cells to allow for faster neural communication. As we get older, our brain is affected by natural signs of aging which can lead to the destruction of neural cells and neurodegenerative diseases like Alzheimer's, dementia, and Parkinson's. The omega-3 fatty acids of the Mediterranean diet are loaded with substances to protect the brain from premature aging and decline in functioning. Along with healthy fruits and vegetables, and removing processed foods and sugars from your diet, you can improve your memory recall, mental focus, and overall cognitive functioning.

Reduces your risk of having type-2 diabetes. For people who have a family history of diabetes or who struggle with unstable blood sugar levels, this type of diabetes can feel imminent in their future. But the Mediterranean diet has been able to lessen the chances of acquiring diabetes (Type 2) because of its healthy eating patterns and allowing you to lose extra weight. Studies have shown that patients can lose more weight following the Mediterranean diet than other low Carb or low-fat diet plans. This is a great way to reduce your risk of diabetes because extra weight is always a risk factor. Patients have seen improvements in their blood sugar levels and even been able to change their medication dosage or quit it entirely! This diet encourages the consumption of fibrous foods like whole grains, beans, legumes, and fresh vegetables. When the body has enough fiber, it's able to slow digestion and make you feel full for a longer period of time. This minimizes the need for frequent snacking which is what can cause blood sugar spikes every time you eat. This means less insulin is produced. The Mediterranean diet doesn't follow a low carbohydrate philosophy, but it cuts foods that cause blood sugar spikes from your diet such as sugary snacks, refined grains, and soda.

Maintains bone density and overall agility of the body as you age. As we age, especially women, in particular, we lose bone density and muscle mass at an alarming speed. Recent research has found that when people who were over the age of 55 years followed the Mediterranean diet for a period of their life, they were able to have a higher level of bone mass and muscle mass compared to women who ate a diet consisting of red meat. It's important to note that for the Mediterranean diet to give these benefits, it has to be followed earlier than when menopause begins in most women. You cannot expect to only follow it for a few months and gain the benefits. It is a complete lifestyle change that you have to immerse yourself in so that you can feel confident in achieving the health successes further in your life. Whether it's the healthy fats that the Mediterranean diet brings to your diet, like the olive oil and fish, it protects the body and cushions the joints against aging, almost like lubrication.

Could help fight against cancer. There is a lot of research yet to cover in the area of cancer prevention, but some tentative research has labeled the Mediterranean diet as one of the best environments to combat cancer cells. A 2013 Italian research study found that the Mediterranean diet provided the highest levels of fiber, antioxidants, and omega 3 fatty acids compared to other diets. With the high intake of fruits, olive oil, fish, whole grains, vegetables, and wine, you're eating healthier, natural foods and avoiding the garbage of processed foods, trans fats, and sugar. It's important to note that diet only goes so far, and this information is in the very early stages. You should always go for cancer screenings and annual health exams.

Can improve your digestive functioning and health. With a diet high in fiber from whole grains, fruits, and vegetables, it's no wonder the Mediterranean diet can help ease any digestive issues! Some diets make you constipated as they cut ingredients out of your diet or reduce the intake of fiber drastically. With the Mediterranean diet focused on plant-based foods, it provides the body with healthy vitamins, minerals, and fiber. Studies have shown that those who consume predominantly meat had a lower variety of gut bacteria. Having more gut bacteria is essential for promoting digestive health and ensuring regular bowel movements to remove waste. Studies have shown that the more frequently your body expels waste, the less risk of developing colon cancer.

Could lower the risk of mental illnesses like depression and anxiety. Other areas where more research is necessary is in mental illnesses. Some research has linked depression, obsessive-compulsive disorder, and anxiety to high amounts of inflammation in the body. With the Mediterranean diet, you're eating high-quality foods that prevent inflammation. Fish and plant-based foods, in particular, have great anti-inflammatory properties, as well as the wine you're encouraged to drink in moderation.

Can clear acne breakouts and improve the look and health of your skin. Any dermatologist will tell you that sugar is bad for your skin and can cause pimples or acne breakouts. Not only that, but it can also destroy the natural collagen present under your skin which is what gives skin that youthful elasticity. The Mediterranean diet can help skin health two-fold: by having a diet rich in fruits and vegetables with natural antioxidants to keep the skin healthy, and by avoiding processed sugar that is found in baked goods and candy. The natural sugars found in fruit are not harmful to the body compared to refined sugar which can cause blood sugar spikes followed by skin irritations. Studies have found that when adult women who did not consume enough fish or fresh fruits and vegetables a week had nearly double the risk of having adult acne.

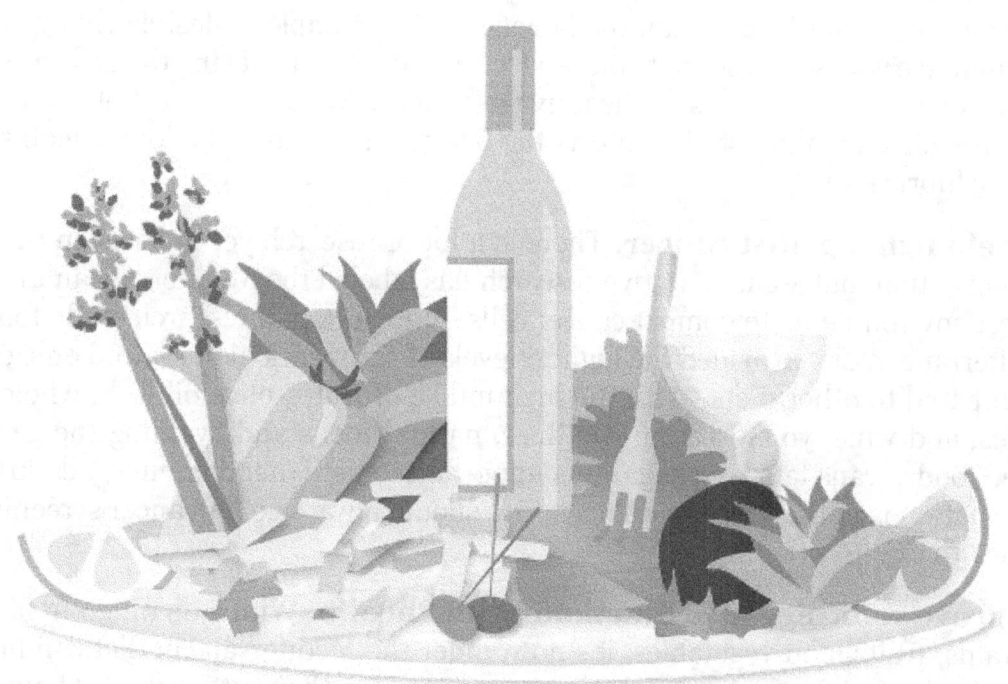

CHAPTER 4: WHY THE MEDITERRANEAN DIET?

There is no calorie-counting! This is one of those positives that people love about the Mediterranean diet. So many new diets restrict people on a calorie basis which can be quite frustrating and often detrimental to your health if you require a greater caloric intake for your physical and health needs. If you're required to count calories, you must be very careful to remember every little thing you're eating as a snack, or even adding on your dishes like dressing or cheese. The Mediterranean diet offers a great amount of flexibility regarding this because it's shifting you away from unhealthy food choices to healthier ones. Of course, you should be aware of your dietary choices and avoid overeating, but you also have the freedom to decide on your portion sizes which means you can take an extra few veggies if you'd like, or you can skip having a snack if you're not feeling hungry. The idea is to eat more filling meals that will ensure you aren't feeling hungry other than at mealtimes. By cutting out the sugar, junk food, and fast food from your diet and loading up on fiber from fruits, vegetables, and whole grains, you're eating healthier without having to worry about every item's calorie count.

You can have wine! If you're someone who already enjoys a glass of wine to unwind after a long day, this is going to be an aspect you love about the Mediterranean diet. You get to have that glass of wine and feel good that it is allowed on your diet and can have heart-healthy properties. Recent research on red wine has found that it is high in antioxidants that may prevent cardiovascular heart disease. The people of the Mediterranean also enjoyed having red wine with a meal so it could tentatively be linked to their excellent cardiovascular health. But it's important to note many warnings regarding alcohol consumption. The Mediterranean diet encourages "moderate consumption," which means there are limits in place. Healthy men can drink 2 glasses a day. Healthy women may have up to 1 glass a day. Also, these possible health benefits are only associated with red wine - not other alcoholic beverages or hard liquor. If you're an avid drinker of those and hoping to substitute that for wine in your Mediterranean diet, that won't work! Before incorporating alcohol into your diet, you should speak to your doctor to ensure it does not interfere with your health, family history, if you're pregnant or breastfeeding, or any medication you may be taking.

You don't have to be drinking wine to gain the benefits of the diet, but if you are a drinker, then you're going to love this diet even more!

The Mediterranean diet is full of fiber-rich foods so you will feel full for longer. Some diets will often restrict the number of carbohydrates, fruit, or vegetable that you can eat due to worries about too much glucose production from carbs, or natural sugars contained in fruit. Thankfully, the Mediterranean diet does no such thing! And that's a good thing because it allows you to have a diet full of fibrous foods. Beans, whole grains, lentils, and fresh vegetables are rich in fiber which is great for your body. Fiber keeps you feeling full for a longer period which means you are less likely to snack in between meals. That means fewer calories and more weight loss! Not only that, but some diets can also have a damaging effect on your digestive system causing constipation or diarrhea due to changes in your regular fiber intake. With the Mediterranean diet, having this high intake of fiber will keep your digestive tract functioning smoothly and keep your bowel movements regular. That means less chance of gastrointestinal or rectal problems. Fiber also gives you energy which is why many people will try and have whole grains for breakfast, such as whole-grain cereal, whole wheat bread, or whole-grain oatmeal.

This diet will improve your mental alertness. The Mediterranean diet removes all the processed and unhealthy substances from your diet such as refined grains, soda, fast food, trans fats, and junk food. That can be tough to do, but the results it brings are very beneficial for your body and mind. All these sugary treats would cause spikes in your blood sugar and cause a rush of insulin throughout the body. That brings around symptoms like mood swings, false hunger pants, irritability, fatigue, and weakness. Instead of keeping you mentally alert, those foods slow you down and distract you from working at your best potential. When following the Mediterranean diet, you are replacing the processed sugars with fresh vegetables and fruits that are full of healthy minerals like vitamin B, folic acid, potassium, vitamin D, omega 3 fatty acids, and more! This keeps the body functioning in top mental and cognitive functioning which gives you more alertness, focus, memory recall, and concentration.

You can have fruit, which is great to satisfy your sweet tooth! Many diets forbid you from eating fruit because of their natural sugars and the net carbs that they could add to your daily caloric intake. This can be quite tough, especially if you're already giving up artificial and refined sugar. Sometimes, your sweet tooth just needs to be satisfied! The more you must give up, often the more tempting it will be to reach for those same ingredients! With the Mediterranean diet, you're encouraged to make fruit a healthy dessert option. Instead of unhealthy sugary snacks, fruit should be your go-to. Whether it's juicy watermelon, a ripe banana, or sweet berries, these natural sugars are much less harmful to your body than artificial ones. Portion size is important, so you don't want to go overboard, but many people are happy to have this option as a sweet treat!

It's very easy to adjust if you're eating outside of your home. One of the worries when you're dieting is feeling constrained if you're ever outside the comfort of your own home at mealtimes. Especially if your diet requires specialized ingredients without a lot of freedom in making meal choices at restaurants or a friend's house. You may be panicking and wondering how to adjust. With the Mediterranean diet, it's very easy to do just that! Let's say you're out at dinner with friends. What can you order that would fit the requirements of the Mediterranean diet? Most places will offer a seafood option so you can have your choice of fish, lobster, shrimp, or crab! If there isn't a seafood choice, you can pick a poultry option - just be sure to avoid red meat! You can also pick a side of fresh vegetables or a small salad. When it comes to dessert, be sure to go for the most natural and organic option instead of a baked good full of refined sugar. You can ask for fresh fruit, or maybe an organic smoothie. The ease and flexibility that the Mediterranean diet allows even when you are outside of the home and away from your prepared meals is what makes it such a favorite among its followers. There's no panic about breaking your diet or making an unhealthy food choice.

There's so much delicious variety to choose from in the Mediterranean diet. This is not a diet you will get bored of easily or feel like the food choice is restricting. There is so much that you can eat and so many foods and recipes you can try. Remember, the Mediterranean region includes countries like Greece, Turkey, Spain, Italy, Morocco, and many more! So, there are always new recipes and ethnic foods that you can include in your menu. Maybe by experimenting, you'll find a new favorite! Not only that, but there are also great varieties of protein that you can incorporate in your dishes, as well as vegetables, whole grains, poultry, and the occasional meal of red meat. You're also encouraged to use spices, fresh herbs, and olive oil to add flavor to your meal which gives it another depth of flavor. With many avenues of exploration, you will not feel constrained by this diet or feel like you're running out of things to eat. Of course, there are clear items you should avoid like trans fats, sugar, and processed foods, but focusing on what you can eat will allow you to enjoy your meals so much more and be excited for the next one!

There will be no harmful side effects that often occur when you reduce your intake of carbohydrates. Many diets lately have been embracing the concept of low carbohydrate intake believing it causes blood sugar spikes and wanting to guide the body through a different fat-burning process called ketosis. The keto diet and other low carb diets drastically reduce the number of carbohydrates you're consuming a day. This can be a quick method to reduce weight, but it can bring a tough adjustment period for the body which includes symptoms like weakness, fatigue, diarrhea, muscle cramps, nausea, and other things that could interfere with your health and daily life. These are temporary, but they could still last a matter of weeks as your body adjusts. That's because carbohydrates tend to make up more than half of our diet. Cutting it down to something very minimal like 5% of your daily intake can be tough on your body! The Mediterranean diet embraces the concept of whole grains because they are healthier for you than refined carbohydrates. They're full of fiber and vitamin B12 and keep you feeling full. Whole grains tend to be lower on the glycemic index compared to refined grains. That means they will not cause blood sugar spikes. This allows you to have a more natural place for whole grains in your diet and still feel confident that you are gaining the health benefits they provide. Cutting something completely from your diet, especially something you will encounter all the time in your food choices, can be very tough and make them seem more tempting!

You don't have to become a gym rat! One of the things that people also love about the Mediterranean diet is that it doesn't require intense exercise that some diets will encourage. This makes it appealing to people of all health levels and physical fitness. It simply encourages you to incorporate more physical activity into your routine, whether that's a walk around the block, a swim session at the pool, or jogging or biking. You don't have to join an array of gym classes or feel like you're not doing enough to burn calories. The people of the Mediterranean very naturally fit exercise into their daily life and activities. They didn't end up dreading it or getting burned out which can often happen if you're following a diet where you must devote too much time at the gym. Instead, try and make the choices to be more active voluntarily, such as taking the stairs instead of the elevator, or parking your car a few blocks away and enjoying the walk to work. This way, you're still burning calories which means you're keeping yourself healthy and losing weight at the same time!

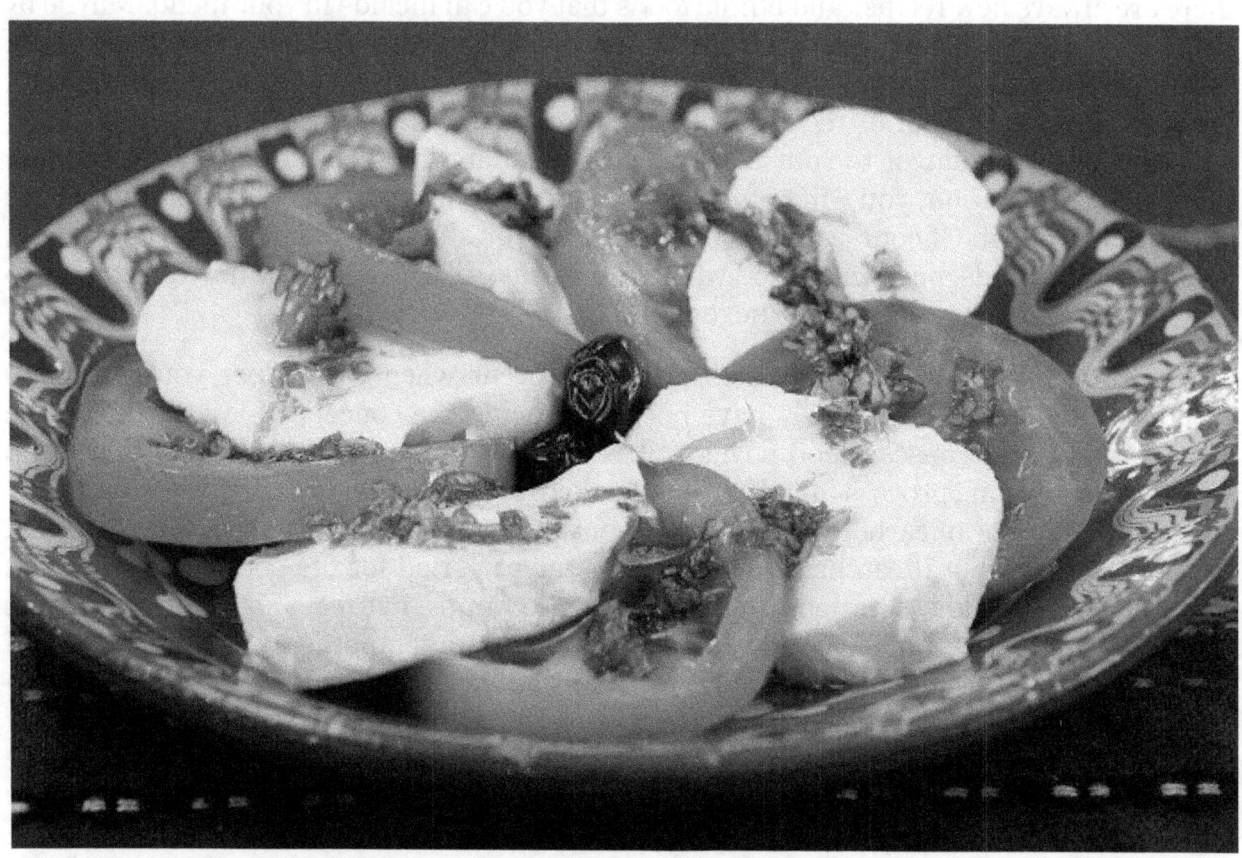

CHAPTER 5: STARTING THE MEDITERRANEAN DIET

The initial step to getting the Mediterranean diet started is to learn its foundations, that is, the ingredients that make it up and make it one of the world's healthiest choices.

1. OLIVE OIL AS A FAT PREFERENCE

Abundant in antioxidants, vitamin E, and fatty acids, the Mediterranean diet's essential oil is olive oil. For example, it is being used to season salads, fry, and toast; all of that needs some form of fat for seasoning or cooking!

So, if you're thinking about starting to go on a Mediterranean diet, leave the butter and eat olive oil.

2. REGULAR INTAKE OF PLANT FOODS

For their significant contribution of antioxidants, fiber, vitamins A and B, minerals, grains, fruits, vegetables, and nuts are eaten every day and regularly. However, according to the Mediterranean diet pyramid, each individual sitting should include one to two pieces of fruits, more than two vegetable servings, natural or cooked, andpreferably, one raw daily portion.

3. DAILY CEREAL CONSUMPTION

1 or 2 portions of cereal are recommended per meal, preferably whole grain in the form of couscous, bread, pasta, rice, etc. The carbohydrates derived out of the given foods will, of course, provide the necessary energy to face the day.

4. CHOOSE FRESH, SEASONAL FOODS

The purchase and use of fresh and seasonal foods allows us to enjoy their nutrients, taste, and fragrance. Use produce thatis unprocessed and in season. It is a safe step and is environmentally friendly.

5. MODERATE CONSUMPTION OF RED MEAT

Because of the health problems that animal fat intake can create, moderate consumption of red and processed meat is recommended. Therefore, according to the Mediterranean diet, the saturated fats of these meats must be reduced.

6. DAILY CONSUMPTION OF DAIRY PRODUCTS
Cheese and yogurt are a staple every day in the Med diet and contain important nutrients such as proteins, vitamins, phosphorus, and calcium.

7. INCREASED CONSUMPTION OF FISH AND EGGS
Starting the Med diet, it's important to reduce your consumption of pork, lamb, and beef or any kind of reddish meat. Instead, you should consume fish and seafood (for its content of Omega-3 fatty acids) and eggs (as a source of quality protein).

8. VERY LOW CONSUMPTIONS OF BAKERY AND SWEET PRODUCTS
It's not a matter of removing these ingredients from your diet entirely but note that your consumption should be extremely moderate. Actually, it is recommended thatyou consume fewer than 2 plates of bakery and sweet products in 7 days.

9. WATER AS A PREFERRED DRINK
Water is a key Mediterranean diet pillar and is essential as a favorite drink. Furthermore, wine can also be consumed in moderation and usual fashion.

10. PHYSICAL EXERCISE
A great diet is one of the best ways to be healthy but isn't the only way to be in great shape. Therefore, make sure to exercise daily and regularly to enjoy the benefits of a healthy diet.

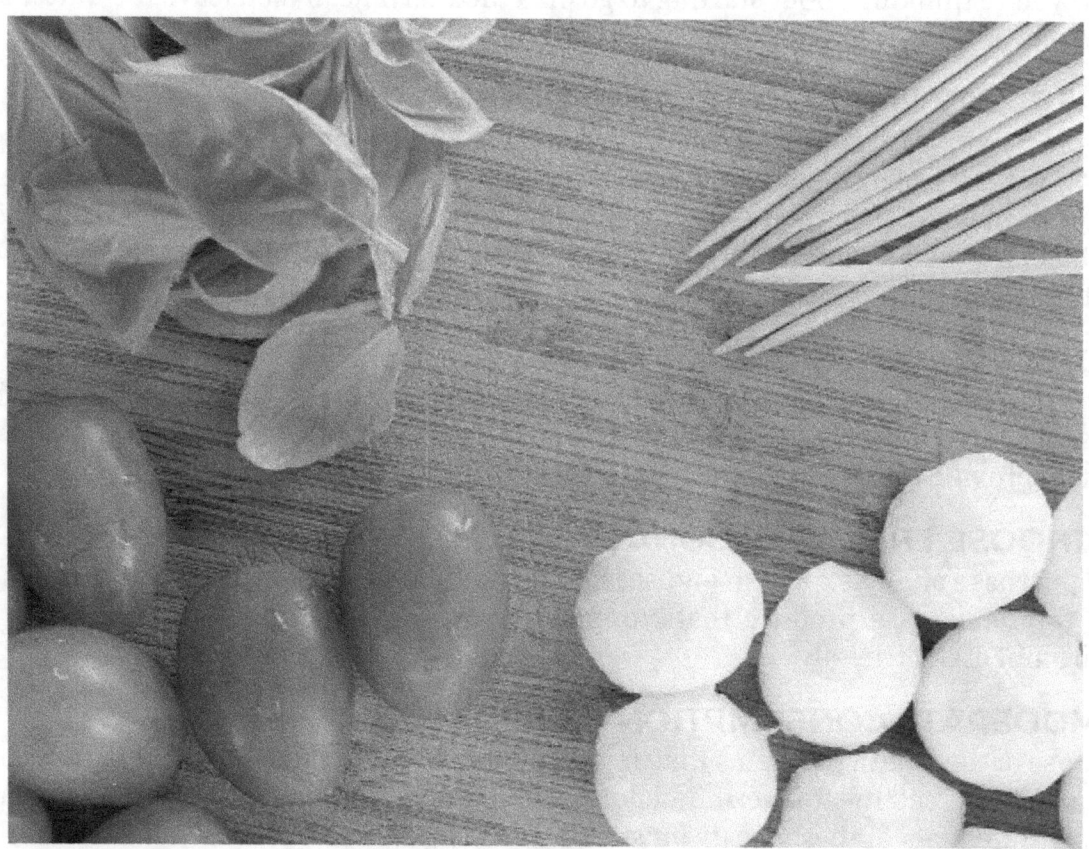

CHAPTER 6: MEDITERRANEAN DIET FOOD PYRAMID

The Mediterranean diet food pyramid is a nutrition guide to help people eat the right foods in the correct quantities and the prescribed frequency as per the traditional eating habits of people from the Mediterranean coast countries.

The pyramid was developed by the World Health Organization, Harvard School of Public Health, and the Oldways Preservation Trust in 1993.

There are 6 food layers in the pyramid with physical activity at the base, which is an important element to maintain a healthy life.

Just above it is the first food layer, consisting of whole grains, bread, beans, pasta, and nuts. It is the strongest layer, with foods that are recommended by the Mediterranean diet. Next comes fruits and vegetables. As you move up the pyramid, you will find foods that must be eaten less and less, with the topmost layer consisting of foods that should be avoided or restricted.

The Mediterranean diet food pyramid is easy to understand. It provides an easy way to follow the eating plan.

The Food Layers: Whole Grains, Bread, Beans – The lowest and the widest layer with foods that are strongly recommended. Your meals should be made of mostly these items. Eat whole-wheat bread, whole-wheat pita, whole-grain roll and bun, whole-grain cereal, whole-wheat pasta, and brown rice. 4 to 6 servings a day will give you plenty of nutrition.

Fruits, Vegetables – Almost as important as the lowest layer. Eat non-starchy vegetables daily like asparagus, broccoli, beets, tomatoes, carrots, cucumber, cabbage, cauliflower, turnips 4 to 8 servings daily. Take 2 to 4 servings of fruits every day. Choose seasonal fresh fruits.

Olive oil – Cook your meals preferably in extra-virgin olive oil. Daily consumption. Healthy for the body, it lowers the low-density lipoprotein cholesterol (LDL) and total cholesterol level. Up to 2 tablespoons of olive oil are allowed. The diet also allows for canola oil.

Poultry, cheese, yogurt – The diet should include cheese, yogurt, eggs, chicken, and other poultry products, but in moderation. Maximum 2-3 times in a week. Low-fat dairy is preferable. Soymilk, cheese, or yogurt is best.

Meats, sweets – This is the topmost layer consisting of foods that are best avoided. You can have red meat once or twice in a week, sweets only once a month. Remember, the Mediterranean diet is plant-based. There is very little room for meat, especially red meat. If you cannot live without it, then take red meat in small portions. Choose lean cuts. Have sweets only to celebrate. For instance, you can have a couple of sweets after following the diet for a month.

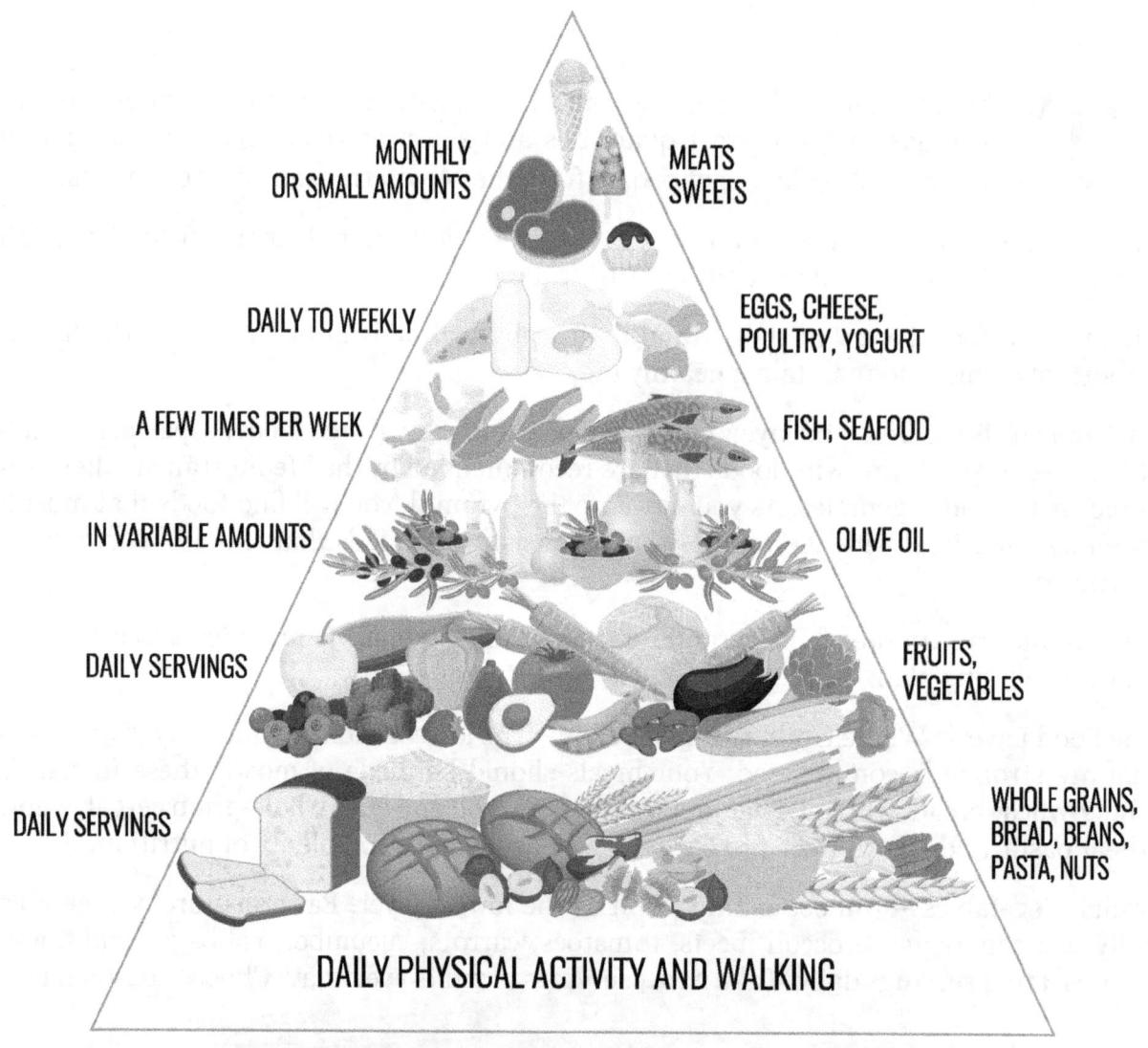

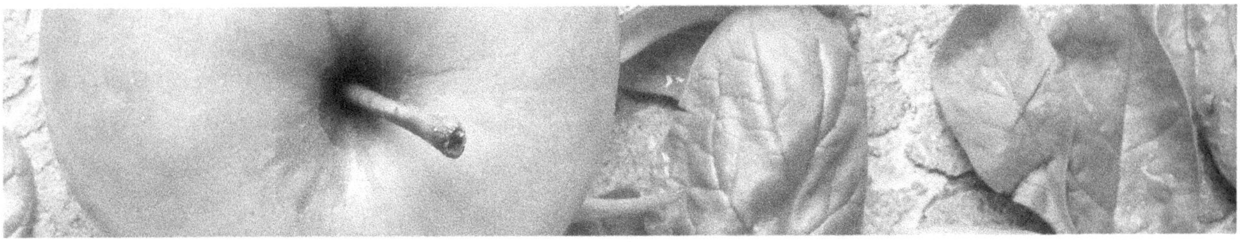

CHAPTER 7:
Smoothie Recipes

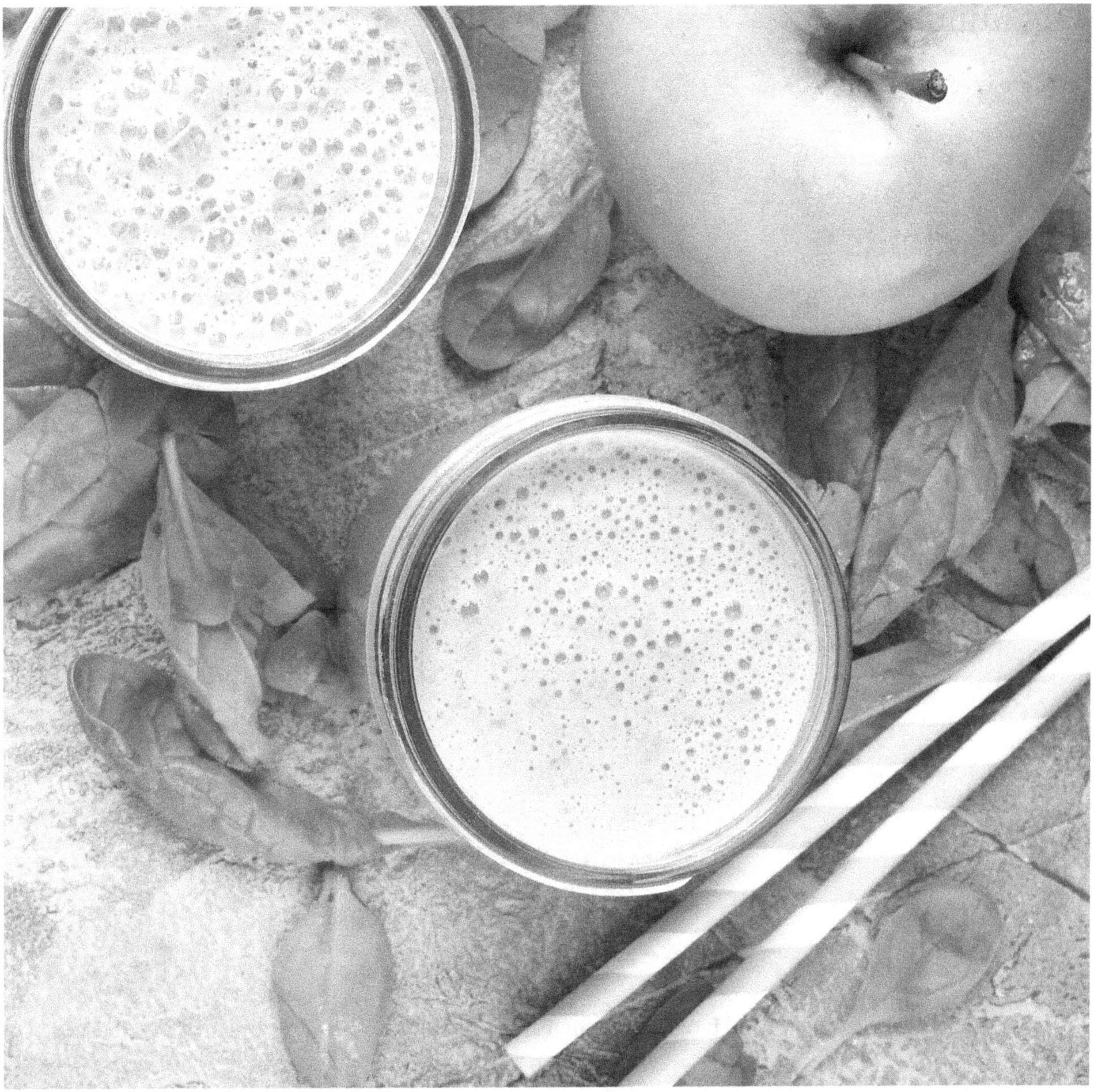

1. Sweet Kale Smoothie

Preparation:
10 Minutes

Cooking:
15 Minutes

Servings:
2

Directions

1. In a blender, combine the yogurt, apple juice, apple, and dates and pulse until smooth.
2. Add the kale and lemon juice and pulse until blended. Add the ice cubes and blend until smooth and thick. Pour into glasses and serve.

Ingredients

- 1 cup low-fat plain Greek yogurt
- ½ cup apple juice
- 1 apple, cored and quartered
- 4 Medjool dates
- 3 cups packed coarsely chopped kale
- Juice of ½ lemon
- 4 ice cubes

Nutritions: Calories: 355, Total fat: 2g, Saturated fat: 1g, Carbohydrates: 77g, Sugar: 58g, Fiber: 8g, Protein: 11g

2. Cranberry-Pumpkin Smoothie

Preparation: 5 Minutes

Cooking: 0 Minutes

Servings: 2

Directions

1. In a blender, combine the almond milk, pumpkin, oats, cranberry juice, honey, cinnamon, and nutmeg and blend until smooth.
2. Pour into glasses and serve immediately.

Ingredients

- 2 cups unsweetened almond milk
- 1 cup pure pumpkin purée
- ¼ cup gluten-free rolled oats
- ¼ cup pure cranberry juice (no sugar added)
- 1 tablespoon honey
- ¼ teaspoon ground cinnamon
- Pinch of ground nutmeg

Nutritions: *Calories: 190, Total fat: 7g, Saturated fat: 0g, Carbohydrates: 26g, Sugar: 12g, Fiber: 5g, Protein: 4g*

3. Chocolate Banana Smoothie

Preparation:
5 Minutes

Cooking:
0 Minutes

Servings:
2

Directions

1. In a blender, combine the bananas, almond milk, ice, cocoa powder, and honey. Blend until smooth.

Ingredients

- 2 bananas, peeled
- 1 cup unsweetened almond milk, or skim milk
- 1 cup crushed ice
- 3 tablespoons unsweetened cocoa powder
- 3 tablespoons honey

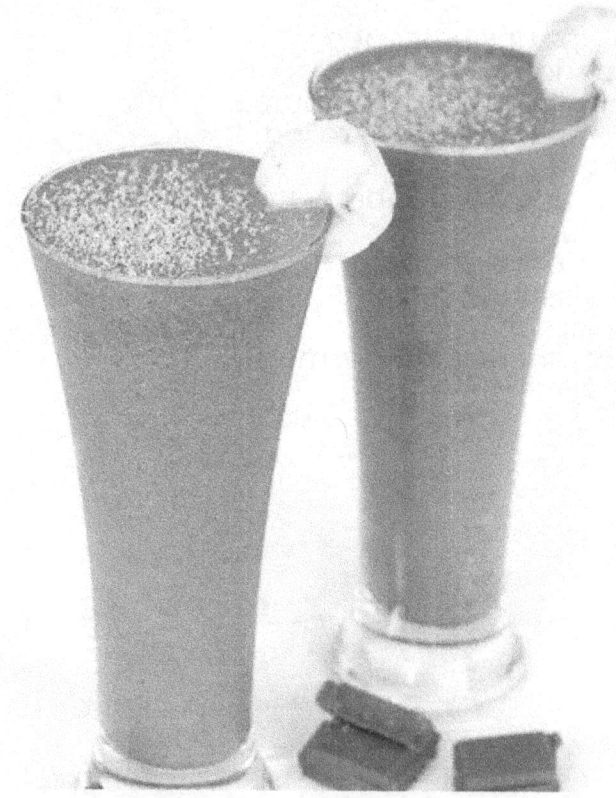

Nutritions: Calories: 219, Protein: 2g, Total Carbohydrates: 57g, Sugars: 40g, Fiber: 6g, Total Fat: 2g, Saturated, Fat: <1g, Cholesterol: 0mg, Sodium: 4mg

4. Fruit Smoothie

Preparation:
5 Minutes

Cooking:
0 Minutes

Servings:
2

Directions

1. 2 cups blueberries (or any fresh or frozen fruit, cut into pieces if the fruit is large)
2. 2 cups unsweetened almond milk
3. 1 cup crushed ice
4. ½ teaspoon ground ginger (or other dried ground spice such as turmeric, cinnamon, or nutmeg)

Ingredients

- In a blender, combine the blueberries, almond milk, ice, and ginger. Blend until smooth.

Nutritions: *Calories: 125, Protein: 2g, Total Carbohydrates: 23g, Sugars: 14g, Fiber: 5g, Total Fat: 4g, Fat: <1g, Cholesterol: 0mg, Sodium: 181mg*

5. Mango-Pear Smoothie

Preparation: 10 Minutes

Cooking: 0 Minutes

Servings: 1

Directions

1. In a blender, purée the pear, mango, kale, and yogurt.
2. Add the ice and blend until thick and smooth. Pour the smoothie into a glass and serve cold.

Ingredients

- 1 ripe pear, cored and chopped
- ½ mango, peeled, pitted, and chopped
- 1 cup chopped kale
- ½ cup plain Greek yogurt
- 2 ice cubes

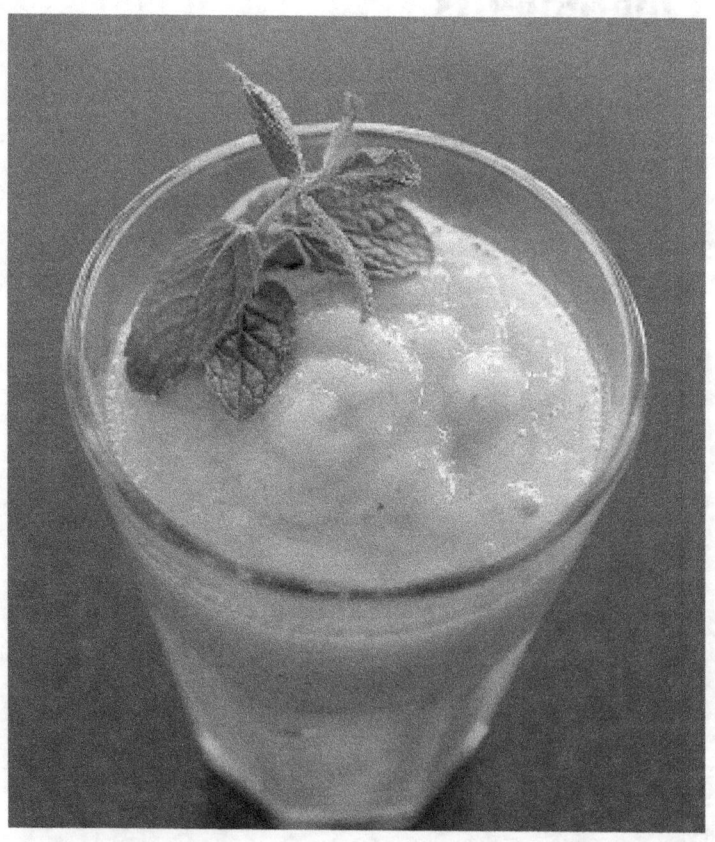

Nutritions: Calories: 293, Total Fat: 8g, Saturated Fat: 5g, Carbohydrates: 53g, Fiber: 7g, Protein: 8g

6. Avocado-Blueberry Smoothie

Preparation: 5 Minutes

Cooking: 0 Minutes

Servings: 2

Directions

1. In a blender, combine the almond milk, yogurt, avocado, blueberries, oats, and vanilla and pulse until well blended.
2. Add the ice cubes and blend until thick and smooth. Serve.

Ingredients

- ½ cup unsweetened vanilla almond milk
- ½ cup low-fat plain Greek yogurt
- 1 ripe avocado, peeled, pitted, and coarsely chopped
- 1 cup blueberries
- ¼ cup gluten-free rolled oats
- ½ teaspoon vanilla extract
- 4 ice cubes

Nutritions: *Calories: 273, Total fat: 15g, Saturated fat: 2g, Carbohydrates: 28g, Sugar: 10g, Fiber: 9g, Protein: 10g*

7. Blueberry Banana Protein Smoothie

Preparation:
5 Minutes

Cooking:
5 Minutes

Servings:
1

Directions

1. Add all of the ingredients into an instant pot ace blender.
2. Blend until smooth.

Ingredients

- ½ cup frozen and unsweetened blueberries
- ½ banana slices up
- ¾ cup plain nonfat Greek yogurt
- ¾ cup unsweetened vanilla almond milk
- 2 cups of ice cubes

Nutritions: Calories: 230, Protein: 19.1g, Total Fat: 2.6g, Carbohydrates: 32.9g

8. Honey and Wild Blueberry Smoothie

Preparation:
5 Minutes

Cooking:
10 Minutes

Servings:
2

Directions

1. Add all of the above ingredients into an Instant Pot Ace blender. Add extra ice cubes if needed.
2. Process until smooth.

Ingredients

- 1 whole banana
- 1 cup of mango chunks
- ½ cup wild blueberries
- ½ plain, nonfat Greek yogurt
- ½ cup milk (for blending)
- 1 tablespoon raw honey
- ½ cup of kale

Nutritions: *Calories: 223, Protein: 9.4g, Total Fat: 1.4g, Carbohydrates: 46.8g*

9. Oats Berry Smoothie

Preparation:
5 Minutes

Cooking:
5 Minutes

Servings:
2

Directions

1. In a blender, combine the yogurt, apple juice, apple, and dates and pulse until smooth.
2. Add the kale and lemon juice and pulse until blended. Add the ice cubes and blend until smooth and thick. Pour into glasses and serve.

Ingredients

- 1 cup of frozen berries
- 1 cup Greek yogurt
- ¼ cup of milk
- ¼ cup of oats
- 2 teaspoon honey

Nutritions: Calories: 295, Protein: 18g, Total Fat: 5g, Carbohydrates: 44g

10. Hearty Pear and Mango Smoothie

Preparation:
10 Minutes

Cooking:
0 Minutes

Servings:
1

Directions

1. Add pear, mango, yogurt, kale, and mango to a blender and puree.
2. Add ice and blend until you have a smooth texture.
3. Serve and enjoy!

Ingredients

- 1 ripe mango, cored and chopped
- ½ mango, peeled, pitted, and chopped
- 1 cup kale, chopped
- ½ cup plain Greek yogurt
- 2 ice cubes

Nutritions: *Calories: 293, Fat: 8g, Carbohydrates: 53g, Protein: 8g*

11. Fig Smoothie with Cinnamon

Preparation:
5 Minutes

Cooking:
10 Minutes

Servings:
2

Directions

1. In a blender, combine the yogurt, apple juice, apple, and dates and pulse until smooth.
2. Add the kale and lemon juice and pulse until blended. Add the ice cubes and blend until smooth and thick. Pour into glasses and serve.

Ingredients

- 3 dessertspoons porridge oats
- 1 large ripe fig
- 6 ¾ oz. orange juice
- 3 rounded dessertspoons Greek yogurt
- ½ teaspoon ground cinnamon
- 3 ice cubes

Nutritions: Calories: 355, Total fat: 2g, Saturated fat: 1g, Carbohydrates: 77g, Sugar: 58g, Fiber: 8g, Protein: 11g

12. Raspberry Vanilla Smoothie

Preparation:
5 Minutes

Cooking:
5 Minutes

Servings:
2

Directions

1. Take all of your ingredients and place them in an instant pot Ace blender.
2. Process until smooth and liquified.

Ingredients

- 1 cup frozen raspberries
- 6-ounce container of vanilla Greek yogurt
- ½ cup of unsweetened vanilla almond milk

Nutritions: *Calories: 155, Protein: 7g, Total Fat: 2g, Carbohydrates: 30g*

13. Kale-Pineapple Smoothie

Preparation:
5 Minutes

Cooking:
5 Minutes

Servings:
2

Directions

1. Cut the ends off of the cucumbers and then cut the whole cucumber into small cubes. Strip the mint leaves from the stems.
2. Add all of the ingredients to your instant pot Ace blender and blend until smooth.

Ingredients

- 1 Persian cucumber
- fresh mint
- 1 cup of coconut milk
- 1 tablespoon honey
- 1 ½ cups of pineapple pieces
- ¼ pound baby kale

Nutritions: Calories: 140, Protein: 4g, Total Fat: 2.5g, Carbohydrates: 30g

CHAPTER 8:
Breakfast Recipes

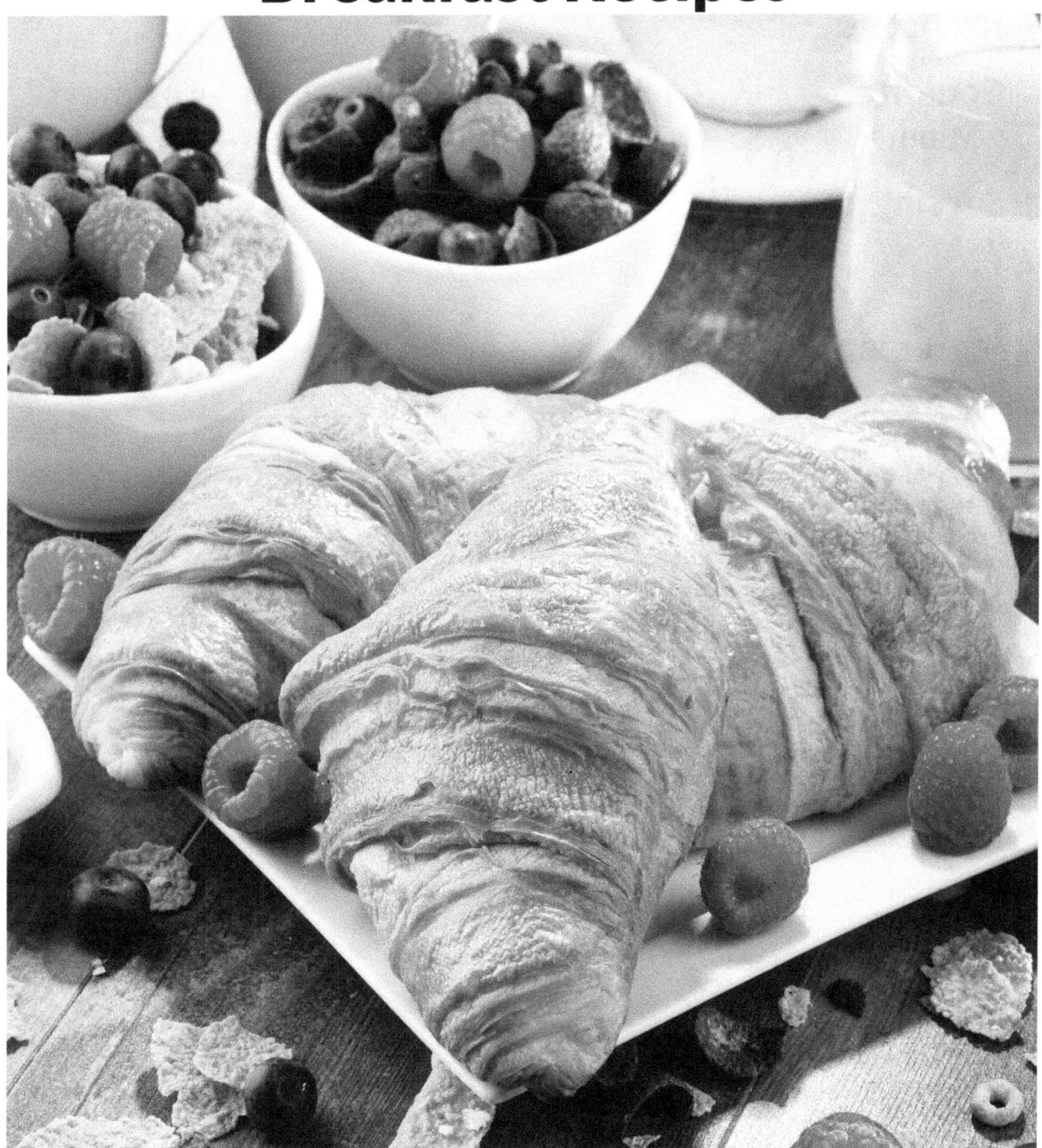

14. Greek Bowl

Preparation:
10 Minutes

Cooking:
7 Minutes

Servings:
7

Directions

1. Boil the eggs in the water for 7 minutes. Then cool them in cold water and peel.
2. Chop the eggs roughly and put them in the salad bowl.
3. Add Greek yogurt, ground black pepper, salt, avocado oil, tomatoes, quinoa, cilantro, and red onion.
4. Shake the mixture well. Serve.

Ingredients

- ¼ cup Greek yogurt
- 12 eggs
- ¼ teaspoon ground black pepper
- ½ teaspoon salt
- 1 tablespoon avocado oil
- 1 cup cherry tomatoes, chopped
- 1 cup quinoa, cooked
- 1 cup fresh cilantro, chopped
- 1 red onion, sliced

Nutritions: Calories: 253, Protein: 16.2g, Carbohydrates: 22.4g, Fat: 11g, Fiber: 2.9g

15. Morning Oats

Preparation:
5 Minutes

Cooking:
0 Minutes

Servings:
2

Directions

1. Mix the ingredients together and leave for 5 minutes.
2. Transfer the meal to the serving bowls.

Ingredients

- 1 oz pecans, chopped
- ¼ cup oats
- ½ cup plain yogurt
- 1 date, chopped
- ½ teaspoon vanilla extract

Nutritions: *Calories: 196, Protein: 6.5g, Carbohydrates: 16.5g, Fat: 11.6g, Fiber: 2.9g*

16. Yogurt with Dates

Preparation:
10 Minutes

Cooking:
0 Minutes

Servings:
4

Directions

1. Mix up all ingredients in the blender and blend until smooth.
2. Pour it into the serving cups.

Ingredients

- 5 dates, pitted, chopped
- 2 cups plain yogurt
- ½ teaspoon vanilla extract
- 4 pecans, chopped

Nutritions: Calories: 215, Protein: 8.7g, Carbohydrates: 18.5g, Fat: 11.5g, Fiber: 2.3g

17. Spinach Frittata

Preparation:
15 Minutes

Cooking:
20 Minutes

Servings:
6

Ingredients

- ¼ cup kalamata olives, pitted and chopped
- 8 eggs, beaten
- 2 cups spinach, chopped
- 1 tablespoon olive oil
- ½ teaspoon chili flakes
- 2 oz Feta, crumbled
- ¼ cup plain yogurt

Directions

1. Brush the pan with olive oil. After this, mix up all remaining ingredients in the mixing bowl, and pour it into the pan.
2. Bake the frittata for 20 minutes at 355F. Serve.

Nutritions: *Calories: 145, Protein: 9.6g, Carbohydrates: 2.3g, Fat: 10.9g, Fiber: 0.4g*

18. Baked Eggs with Parsley

Preparation:
15 Minutes

Cooking:
20 Minutes

Servings:
6

Directions

1. Warm a pan with the oil over medium heat, add all ingredients except eggs and roast them for 5 minutes.
2. Stir the vegetables well and crack the eggs.
3. Transfer the pan with eggs in the preheated ovenat 360F and bake them for 15 minutes.

Ingredients

- 2 green bell peppers, chopped
- 3 tablespoons olive oil
- 1 yellow onion, chopped
- 1 teaspoon sweet paprika
- 6 tomatoes, chopped
- 6 eggs
- ¼ cup parsley, chopped

Nutritions: Calories 167, Protein:0.3g, Carbohydrates: 10.2g, Fat: 11.8g, Fiber: 2.6g

19. Mushroom Casserole

Preparation:
15 Minutes

Cooking:
60 Minutes

Servings:
4

Directions

1. Mix the ingredients together in the casserole mold and cover it with foil.
2. Bake the casserole for 60 minutes at 355F.

Ingredients

- 2 eggs, beaten
- 1 cup mushrooms, sliced
- 2 shallots, chopped
- 1 teaspoon marjoram, dried
- ½ cup artichoke hearts, chopped
- 3 oz cheddar cheese, shredded
- ½ cup plain yogurt

Nutritions: *Calories: 156, Protein: 11.2g, Carbohydrates: 6.2g, Fat: 9.7g, Fiber: 1.3g*

20. Vanilla Pancakes

Preparation:
15 Minutes

Cooking:
15 Minutes

Servings:
2

Directions

1. Heat non-stick skillet well.
2. Mix the ingredients together.
3. Pour the mixture into the skillet in the shape of the pancakes. Cook them for 1 minute per side. Serve.

Ingredients

- 6 ounces plain yogurt
- ½ cup whole-grain flour
- 1 egg, beaten
- 1 teaspoon vanilla extract
- 1 teaspoon baking powder

Nutritions: Calories: 202, Protein: 11.7g, Carbohydrates: 29.4g, Fat: 3.8g, Fiber: 3.7g

21. Savory Egg Galettes

Preparation:
10 Minutes

Cooking:
30 Minutes

Servings:
4

Ingredients

- ¼ cup white onion, diced
- ¼ cup bell pepper, chopped
- ½ teaspoon salt
- 1 teaspoon chili flakes
- 2 tablespoons olive oil
- 1 teaspoon dried dill
- 6 eggs, beaten
- 2 tablespoons plain yogurt

Directions

1. Mix together the onion, bell pepper, salt, and chili flakes in the pan. Add olive oil and dried dill. Sauté the ingredients for 5 minutes.
2. Then pour the beaten eggs into the square baking mold. Add sautéed onion mixture and plain yogurt.
3. Flatten the mixture and bake in the preheated oven at 360F for 20 minutes. Cut the meal into galettes.
4. Serve.

Nutritions: *Calories: 166, Protein: 9g, Carbohydrates: 2.4g, Fat: 13.5g, Fiber: 0.3g*

MEDITERRANEAN DIET COOKBOOK *for beginners*

22. Arugula Frittata

Preparation:
15 Minutes

Cooking:
25 Minutes

Servings:
12

Directions

1. Warm the olive oil in the pan. Mix up eggs with ground black pepper, arugula, and garlic cloves.
2. Add arugula and pour the mixture into the hot pan. Top the egg mixture with mozzarella and transfer to a preheated oven at 360F. Bake the frittata for 20 minutes. Serve.

Ingredients

- 3 garlic cloves, minced
- 1 tablespoon olive oil
- 1 cup fresh arugula, chopped
- 8 eggs, beaten
- 1 teaspoon ground black pepper
- 1 cup mozzarella cheese, shredded

Nutritions: Calories: 61, Protein: 4.5g, Carbohydrates: 0.7g, Fat: 4.5g, Fiber: 0.1g

23. Breakfast Toast

Preparation:
10 Minutes

Cooking:
20 Minutes

Servings:
6

Directions

1. In the mixing bowl, mix up eggs, cream, and ground cinnamon.
2. Add the mashed banana.
3. Coat the bread in the egg mixture. Then heat the olive oil.
4. Put the coated bread in the hot olive oil and roast for 3 minutes per side until light brown.

Ingredients

- 2 eggs, beaten
- ½ cup yogurt
- 1 banana, mashed
- ½ teaspoon ground cinnamon
- 6 whole-grain bread slices
- 1 tablespoon olive oil

Nutritions: *Calories: 153, Protein: 6.2g, Carbohydrates: 19.2g, Fat: 5.6g, Fiber: 2.6g*

24. Artichoke Omelet

Preparation:
5 Minutes

Cooking:
10 Minutes

Servings:
4

Directions

1. Mix the eggs, chopped artichokes, goat cheese, and tomato. Then brush the baking mold with olive oil and pour the mixture inside.
2. Bake the omelet for 10 minutes at 365F. Serve.

Ingredients

- 4 eggs, beaten
- 1 tomato, chopped
- ½ cup artichoke hearts, chopped
- 4 oz goat cheese, crumbled
- 1 tablespoon olive oil

Nutritions: Calories: 61, Protein: 4.5g, Carbohydrates: 0.7g, Fat: 4.5g, Fiber: 0.1g

25. Bell Pepper Frittata

Preparation:
10 Minutes

Cooking:
15 Minutes

Servings:
4

Directions

1. Brush the baking pan with melted olive oil. Then add all remaining ingredients, mix gently and transfer in the preheated to 365F oven. Cook the frittata for 15 minutes.

Ingredients

- 1 cup red bell pepper, chopped
- 1 tablespoon olive oil, melted
- 1 tomato, sliced
- 4 eggs, beaten
- ¼ teaspoon ground black pepper
- ¼ teaspoon salt

Nutritions: *Calories: 105, Protein: 6g, Carbohydrates: 3.3g, Fat: 7.9g, Fiber: 0.6g*

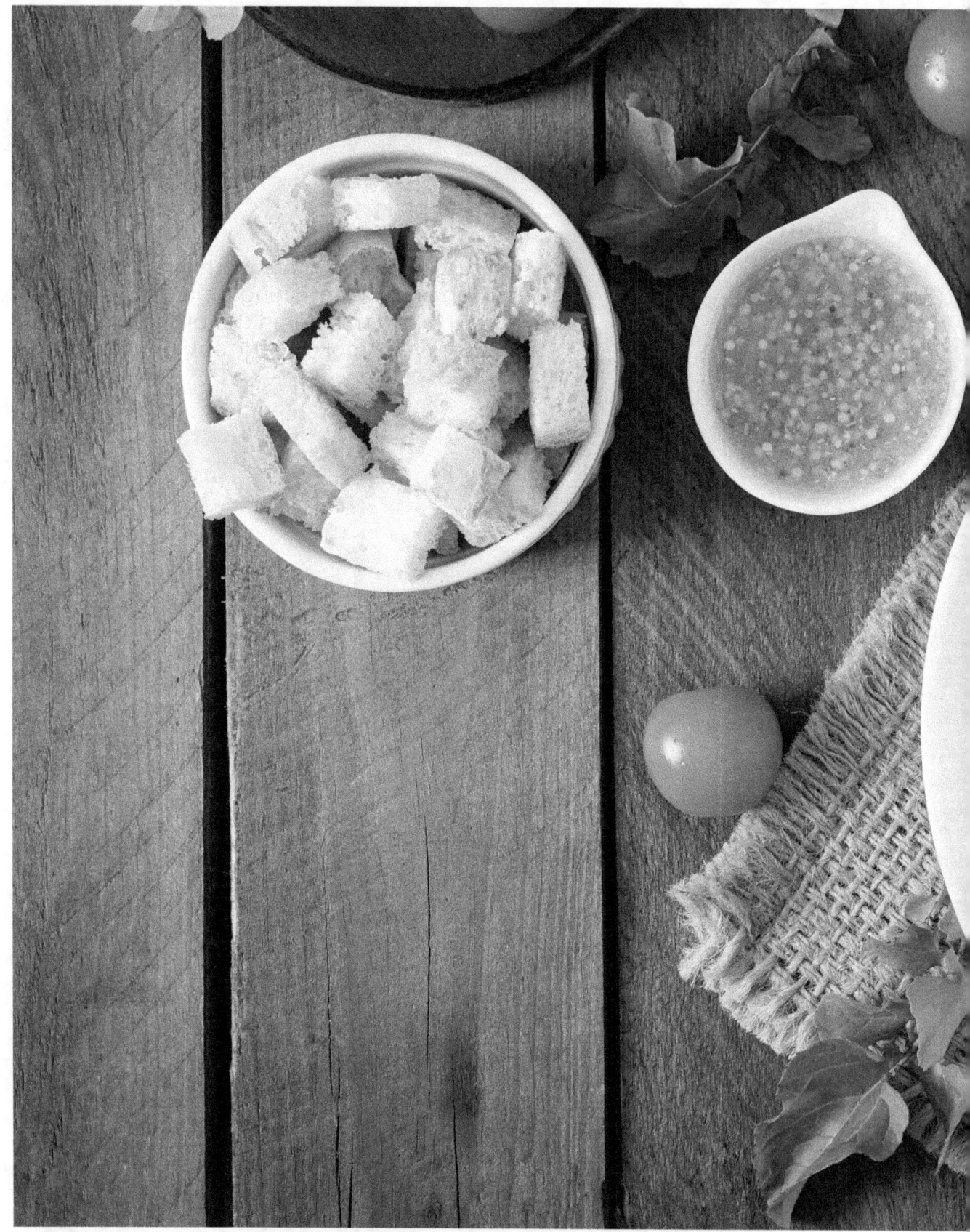

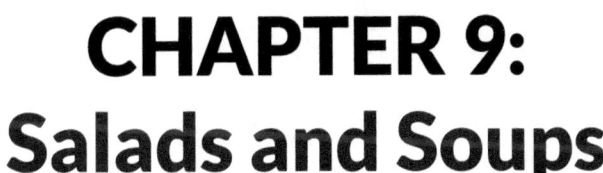

CHAPTER 9:
Salads and Soups

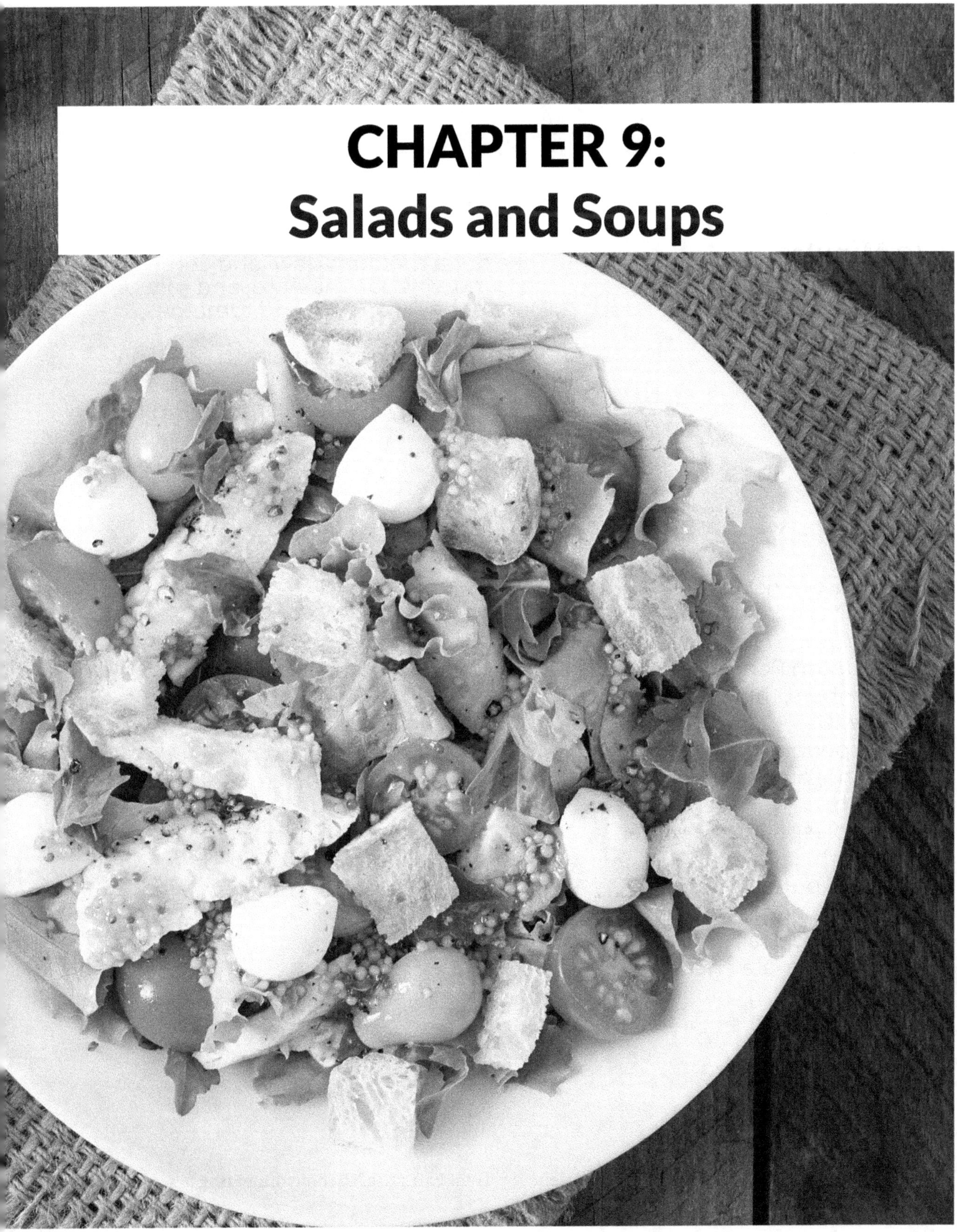

26. Tomato, Cucumber, and Feta Salad

Preparation:
10 Minutes

Cooking:
0 Minutes

Servings:
4

Directions

1. Take out a medium bowl and combine the oregano, vinegar, mustard, and salt.
2. Drizzle the oil on top. Add tomatoes, cucumbers, and feta.
3. Mix them well and serve with oregano leaves as toppings.
4. Refrigerate if you are planning to serve later.

Ingredients

- 3 tablespoons extra-virgin olive oil
- ½ teaspoon Dijon mustard
- 4 medium Persian cucumbers, thinly sliced crosswise
- 1 teaspoon chopped fresh oregano, plus extra for garnish
- 1½ tablespoons red-wine vinegar
- 1 cup (8 ounces) tomatoes, cut into wedges
- ¼ teaspoon salt
- 1½ ounces feta cheese, crumbled

Nutritions: Calories: 153, Protein: 3g, Total Fat: 13.1g, Carbohydrate: 6.1g

27. Goat Cheese Stuffed Tomatoes

Preparation:
10 Minutes

Cooking:
0 Minutes

Servings:
4

Ingredients

- 6-8 arugula leaves
- 3 ounces crumbled feta cheese
- 2 medium ripe tomatoes
- Extra-virgin olive oil to drizzle
- Balsamic vinegar to drizzle
- 1 red onion, very thinly sliced for garnish
- Fresh chopped parsley for garnish
- Salt and freshly ground pepper to taste

Directions

1. Arrange the arugula leaves in the center of a plate.
2. Remove the tops and the core of the tomatoes. Ideally, you should remove the top first and scoop out the core.
3. Fill the tomatoes with feta cheese. Add salt and pepper, to taste
4. Drizzle with olive oil and balsamic vinegar.
5. Garnish with chopped parsley and red onion.
6. Serve at room temperature.

Nutritions: *Calories: 142 calories, Protein: 7g, Total Fat: 13.1g, Carbohydrate: 7g*

28. Classic Tabbouleh

Preparation:
10 Minutes

Cooking:
20 Minutes

Servings:
4

Ingredients

- ¾ cup bulgur
- 2 cups freshly chopped parsley
- 1½ cups water
- ½ cup fresh lemon juice
- ½ cup extra-virgin olive oil
- ½ red bell pepper, diced
- 3 ripe plum tomatoes, peeled, seeded, and diced
- 1 large cucumber, peeled, seeded, and diced
- ¾ cup chopped scallions, white and green parts
- ½ green bell pepper, diced
- ½ cup finely chopped fresh mint
- 1 handful of greens for serving
- Seasoned pita wedges
- Sea salt and freshly ground pepper to taste

Directions

1. Preheat the oven to around 375° F.
2. Take a medium-sized bowl and add the asparagus with 2 tablespoons of salt and olive oil.
3. Take out a baking dish and add the asparagus. Place the tray in the oven and roast for about 10 minutes, or until the asparagus becomes tender.
4. Take out the asparagus and set aside.
5. Use another medium-sized bowl and add garlic, lime juice, orange juice, and the remaining 2 tablespoons of olive oil. Whisk all the ingredients together. Add salt and pepper to taste.
6. Take the lettuce and split it into 6 plates. Take out the asparagus and place it on top of the lettuce.
7. Pour the dressing over the asparagus and lettuce salad. Top the salad with basil and pine nuts. Add a small amount of Romano cheese for garnish.
8. You can also toast the pine nuts in the oven. Use the method below:
9. Take out a baking tray and line it with a non-stick baking sheet. Add the pine nuts on top.
10. Bake at 375 degrees for about 5-10 minutes, or until the nuts are lightly browned.
11. Remove from the oven and set aside to cool.
12. Add the nuts to the salad as a topping.

Nutritions: Calories: 177, Protein: 12g, Total Fat: 11g, Carbohydrate: 28g

MEDITERRANEAN DIET COOKBOOK *for beginners*

29. Mediterranean Greens

Preparation:
10 Minutes

Cooking:
0 Minutes

Servings:
4

Directions

1. Take out a large salad bowl, combine walnuts, greens, tomatoes, onion, and cranberries. Gently toss.
2. For the dressing, combine water, vinegar, oregano, olive oil, and garlic. Mix the ingredients well. Pour over the salad and lightly toss.
3. Add feta cheese as a garnish.
4. Add pepper to taste.

Ingredients

- 6 cups fresh mixed greens (such as radicchio, arugula, watercress, baby spinach, and romaine)
- 1 small red onion, thinly sliced
- 20 cherry tomatoes, halved
- ¼ cup dried cranberries
- ¼ cup chopped walnuts
- Crumbled feta cheese
- Freshly ground pepper to taste
- 2 tablespoons balsamic vinegar
- 2 cloves fresh garlic, finely minced
- 4 tablespoons extra-virgin olive oil
- 1 tablespoon water
- ½ teaspoon crushed dried oregano

Nutritions: *Calories: 140, Protein: 2g, Total Fat: 12g, Carbohydrate: 6g*

30. North African Zucchini Salad

Preparation:
10 Minutes

Cooking:
0 Minutes

Servings:
4

Ingredients

- 1-pound firm green zucchini, thinly sliced
- ½ teaspoon ground cumin
- 2 cloves fresh garlic, finely minced
- Juice from 1 large lemon
- 1 tablespoon extra-virgin olive oil
- 1½ tablespoons plain low-fat yogurt
- Crumbled feta cheese
- Finely chopped parsley for garnish
- Salt and freshly ground pepper to taste

Directions

1. Add the zucchini to a large saucepan and steam it for about 2-5 minutes, or until it becomes tender and crispy. Place the zucchini under cold water and drain well.
2. Take out a large bowl and mix cumin, olive oil, lemon juice, garlic, and yogurt. Add salt and pepper to taste.
3. Add the zucchini to the mixture in the bowl and toss gently.
4. Serve with feta cheese and parsley as garnish.

Nutritions: Calories: 140, Protein: 2g, Total Fat: 12g, Carbohydrate: 6g

31. Avocado Salad

Preparation:
10 Minutes

Cooking:
0 Minutes

Servings:
3

Directions

1. Start with the avocado and cut it into bite-sized pieces.
2. Add parsley, lime juice, tomatoes, onion, and hot pepper. Mix all the ingredients well. Add salt and pepper to taste.
3. Finally, add the avocado into the mixture and mix them well.

Ingredients

- 1 small onion, finely chopped
- 1 large ripe avocado, pitted and peeled
- 2 tablespoons chopped fresh parsley
- 2 teaspoons fresh lime juice
- ½ small hot pepper, finely chopped (optional)
- 1 cup halved cherry tomatoes
- Salt and freshly ground pepper to taste

Nutritions: *Calories: 130, Protein: 2g, Total Fat: 10g, Carbohydrate: 10g*

32. Tunisian Style Carrot Salad

Preparation:
15 Minutes

Cooking:
0 Minutes

Servings:
6

Ingredients

- 10 medium carrots, peeled and sliced
- 1 cup crumbled feta cheese, divided
- 2 teaspoons caraway seed
- ¼ cup extra-virgin olive oil
- 6 tablespoons apple cider vinegar
- 5 teaspoons freshly minced garlic
- 1 tablespoon Harissa paste (choose the level of heat based on your preference)
- 20 pitted Kalamata olives, reserving some for garnish
- Salt to taste

Directions

1. Get a medium saucepan and place it on medium heat. Fill it with water and add the carrots. Cook carrots until tender. Drain and cool the carrots under cold water. Drain again to remove any excess water.
2. Get a large bowl and place the carrots in them.
3. Get a mortar and combine salt, garlic, and caraway seeds. Grind them until they form a paste. Otherwise, you can also use a small bowl to grind, preferably one not made out of glass. The final option would be to toss the ingredients into a blender and pulse them.
4. Add vinegar and Harissa into the bowl with the carrots and mix them well.
5. Use a large spoon and mash the carrots. Add the garlic mixture into the carrot and mix again until they have all blended well. Add the olive oil and mix again.
6. Finally, add about ½ the feta cheese and all the olives and mix well again.
7. Get a large bowl and add the salad to it. Top it with the remaining feta cheese.

Nutritions: Calories: 138 calories, Protein: 7g, Total Fat: 5g, Carbohydrate: 13g

33. Classic Greek Salad

Preparation:
15 Minutes

Cooking:
0 Minutes

Servings:
6

Directions

1. Take out a large bowl and add vinegar, oregano, olive oil, and garlic. Add salt and pepper to taste. Set aside the bowl.
2. In another large bowl, add onion, tomatoes, escarole, cucumber, bell pepper, and cheese and mix them well.
3. Take the vinegar mixture and pour it over the salad in the second bowl.
4. Top the salad with olives and parsley.

Ingredients

- 6 large firm tomatoes, quartered
- 20 Greek black olives
- ½ pound Greek feta cheese, cut into small cubes
- ½ head of escarole, shredded
- 3 tablespoons red wine vinegar
- ¼ cup extra-virgin olive oil
- 1 tablespoon dried oregano
- ½ English cucumber, peeled, seeded, and thinly sliced
- 2 cloves fresh garlic, finely minced
- ½ red onion, sliced
- 1 medium red bell pepper, seeded and sliced
- ¼ cup freshly chopped Italian parsley
- Salt and freshly ground pepper to taste

Nutritions: *Calories: 268 calories, Protein: 23g, Total Fat: 17g, Carbohydrate: 44g*

MEDITERRANEAN DIET COOKBOOK *for beginners*

34. Chicken Leek Soup

Preparation:
10 Minutes

Cooking:
35 Minutes

Servings:
4

Ingredients

- 1 cup cabbage, shredded
- 6 oz leek, chopped
- ½ yellow onion, diced
- 1-pound chicken breast, skinless, boneless
- 1 tablespoon butter
- 1 teaspoon salt
- ½ teaspoon dried oregano
- ½ teaspoon dried thyme
- 1 tablespoon canola oil
- 4 cups of water

Directions

1. Chop the chicken breast into cubes and place it in the pan.
2. Add butter and canola oil.
3. Cook the chicken for 5 minutes. Stir it from time to time.
4. After this, add yellow onion and chopped leek.
5. Add salt, dried oregano, and thyme. Mix up the ingredients well and sauté for 5 minutes.
6. Then add water and cabbage.
7. Close the lid and cook the soup over a medium heat for 25 minutes.

Nutritions: Calories: 222, Fat: 9.4g, Fiber: 1.6g, Carbs: 8.5g, Protein: 25.1g

35. Meatball Soup

Preparation:
10 Minutes

Cooking:
30 Minutes

Servings:
4

Ingredients

- 1 cup ground beef
- 1 tablespoon semolina
- ½ teaspoon salt
- 1 egg yolk
- ½ teaspoon ground black pepper
- 4 cups chicken stock
- 1 carrot, chopped
- 1 yellow onion, diced
- 1 tablespoon butter
- ½ teaspoon turmeric
- ½ teaspoon garlic powder

Directions

1. Toss butter in the skillet and heat it up until it is melted.
2. Add onion and cook it until light brown.
3. Then, pour chicken stock into the pan.
4. Add garlic powder and turmeric.
5. Bring the liquid to boil. Add chopped carrot and boil it for 10 minutes.
6. In the mixing bowl, mix together the ground beef, semolina, salt, egg yolk, and ground black pepper.
7. Make into small-sized meatballs.
8. Put the meatballs in the chicken stock.
9. Add cooked onion.
10. Cook the soup for 15 minutes over a medium-low heat.

Nutritions: *Calories: 143, Fat: 8.8, Fiber: 1.2, Carbs: 7.5, Protein: 8.8*

36. Lemon Lamb Soup

Preparation:
10 Minutes

Cooking:
50 Minutes

Servings:
8

Ingredients

- 1 ½-pound lamb bone-in
- 4 eggs, beaten
- 2 cups lettuce, chopped
- 1 tablespoon chives, chopped
- ½ cup fresh dill, chopped
- ½ cup lemon juice
- 1 teaspoon salt
- ½ teaspoon white pepper
- 2 tablespoons avocado oil
- 5 cups of water

Directions

1. Chop the lamb roughly and place it in the pan.
2. Add avocado oil and roast the meat for 10 minutes over a medium heat. Stir it with the help of a spatula from time to time.
3. Then sprinkle the meat with white pepper and salt. Add water and bring the mixture to boil.
4. In the mixing bowl, whisk together eggs and lemon juice.
5. Add a ½ cup of boiling water from the pan and whisk the egg mixture until smooth.
6. Add dill, chives, and lettuce into the soup. Stir well.
7. Cook the soup for 30 minutes over a medium-high heat.
8. Then add egg mixture and stir it fast to make the homogenous texture of the soup.
9. Cook it for 3 minutes more.

Nutritions: Calories: 360, Fat: 22.9, Fiber: 0.8, Carbs: 2.9, Protein: 33.6

37. Eggplant Soup

Preparation:
10 Minutes

Cooking:
30 Minutes

Servings:
4

Ingredients

- ½ cup tomatoes, chopped
- 2 eggplants, trimmed
- ¼ cup fresh parsley, chopped
- ¼ cup fresh cilantro, chopped
- 1 yellow onion, diced
- ½ teaspoon ground cumin
- ½ teaspoon cayenne pepper
- 1 celery stalk, chopped
- 1 tablespoon olive oil
- 1 teaspoon salt
- 1 garlic clove, peeled
- 1 teaspoon butter
- 4 cups chicken stock

Directions

1. Peel eggplants and sprinkle them with olive oil and salt.
2. Preheat the oven to 360F.
3. Put the eggplants in the tray and transfer it to the preheated oven.
4. Bake the vegetables for 25 minutes.
5. Meanwhile, pour chicken stock into the pan.
6. Add chopped tomatoes, parsley, cilantro, ground cumin, cayenne pepper, celery stalk, and diced garlic clove.
7. Simmer the mixture for 5 minutes.
8. Meanwhile, heat up the butter in the skillet.
9. Add onion and roast it until translucent.
10. Add the onion to the boiled chicken stock mixture.
11. When the eggplants are cooked, transfer them to the food processor and blend until smooth.
12. After this, put the blended eggplants in the chicken stock mixture.
13. Blend the soup with the help of the hand blender until you get a creamy texture.
14. Simmer the soup for 5 minutes.

Nutritions: *Calories: 137, Fat: 5.7, Fiber: 10.9, Carbs: 21.2, Protein: 4.2*

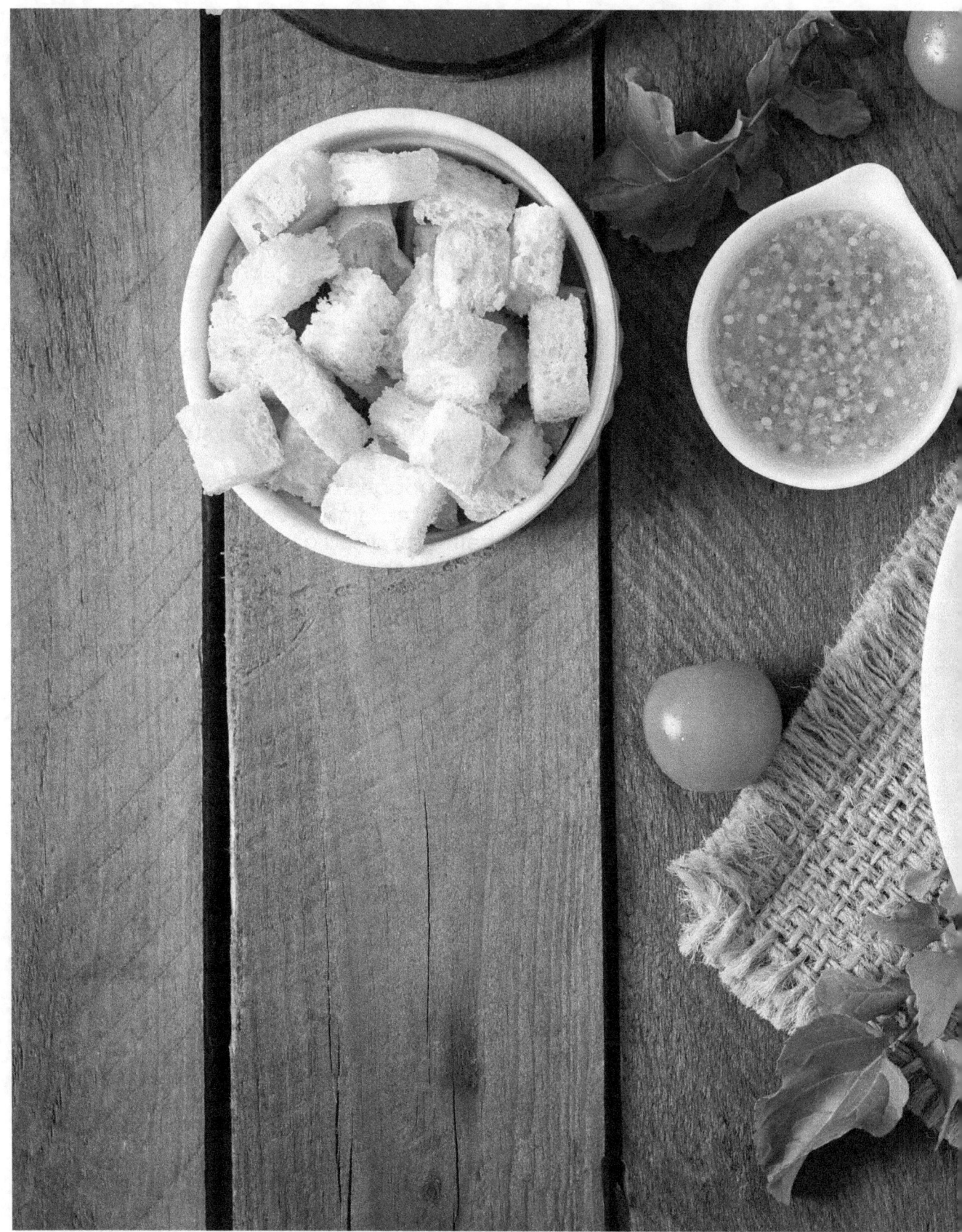

CHAPTER 10:
Pasta, Rice, and Couscous

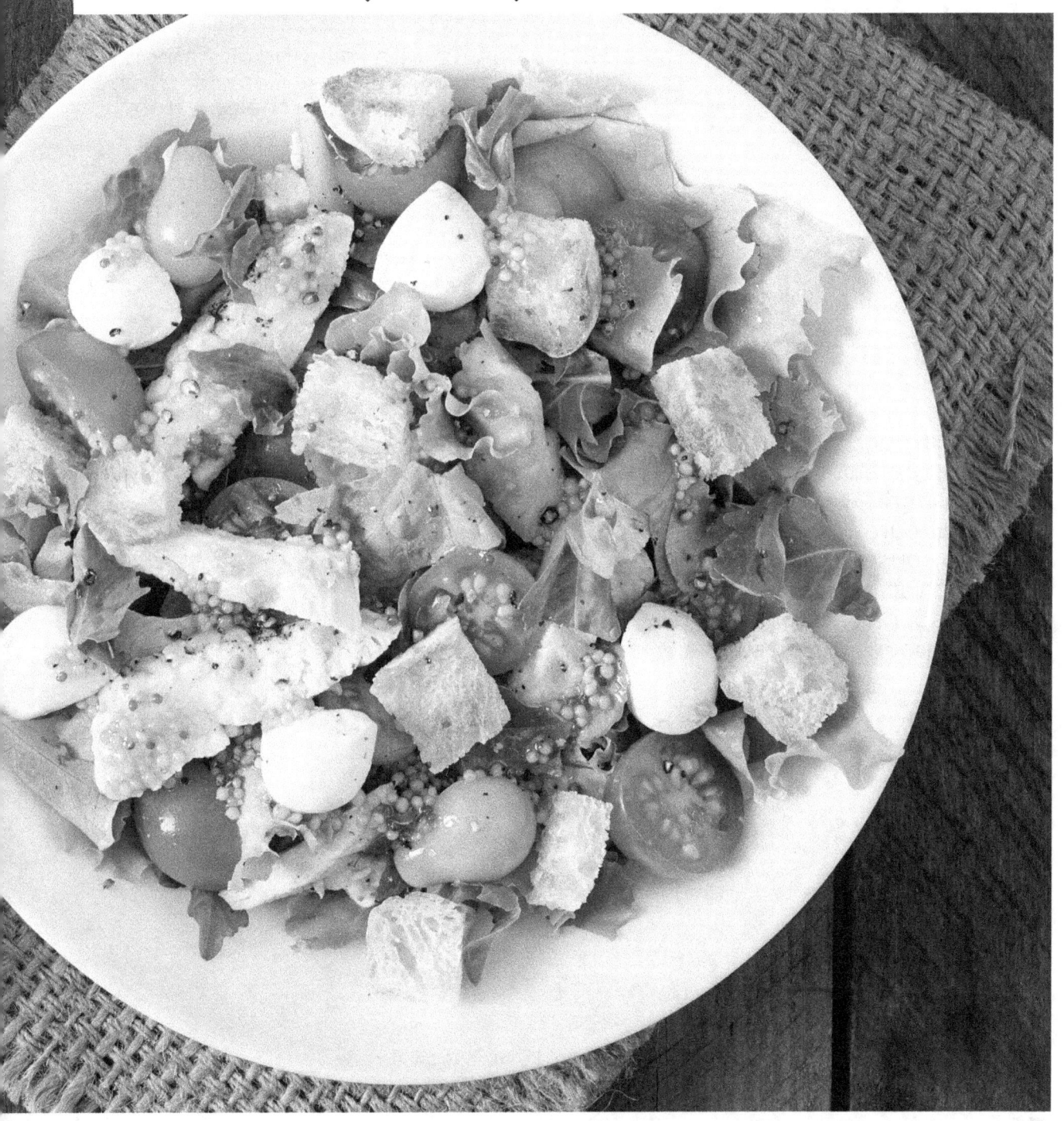

38. Breakfast Couscous

Preparation:
5 Minutes

Cooking:
15 Minutes

Servings:
4

Directions

1. Heat a pan up with milk and cinnamon using medium-high heat. Cook for three minutes before removing the pan from heat.
2. Add in your apricots, couscous, salt, currants, and sugar. Stir well, and then cover. Leave it to the side, and let it sit for fifteen minutes.
3. Remove the cinnamon stick and divide between bowls. Sprinkle with brown sugar before serving.

Ingredients

- 3 cups milk, low fat
- 1 cinnamon stick
- ½ cup apricots, dried & chopped
- ¼ cup currants, dried
- 1 cup couscous, uncooked
- 1 pinch sea salt, fine
- 4 teaspoons butter, melted
- 6 teaspoons brown sugar

Nutritions: Calories: 520, Protein: 39g, Fats: 28g

39. Pork with Couscous

Preparation:
10 Minutes

Cooking:
7 Hours

Servings:
6

Directions

1. In a bowl, mix oil with stock, paprika, garlic powder, sage, rosemary, thyme, marjoram, oregano, salt, and pepper to taste and whisk well. Put pork loin in your Crock-Pot.
2. Add stock and spice mix, stir, cover, and cook on low for 7 hours. Slice pork return to pot and toss with cooking juices.
3. Divide between plates and serve with couscous on the side.

Ingredients

- 2 ½ pounds pork loin, boneless and trimmed
- ¾ cup chicken stock
- 2 tablespoons olive oil
- ½ tablespoon sweet paprika
- 2 ¼ teaspoon sage, dried
- ½ tablespoon garlic powder
- ¼ teaspoon rosemary, dried
- ¼ teaspoon marjoram, dried
- 1 teaspoon basil, dried
- 1 teaspoon oregano, dried
- Salt and black pepper to taste
- 2 cups couscous, cooked

Nutritions: *Calories: 320, Fat: 31, Fiber: 15, Carbs: 21, Protein: 23*

40. Tuna and Couscous

Preparation:
10 Minutes

Cooking:
0 Minutes

Servings:
4

Directions

1. Put the stock in a pan, bring to a boil over medium-high heat, add the couscous, stir, take off the heat, cover, leave aside for 10 minutes, fluff with a fork, and transfer to a bowl.
2. Add the tuna and the rest of the ingredients, toss, and serve for lunch right away.

Ingredients

- 1 cup chicken stock
- 1 ¼ cups couscous
- A pinch of salt and black pepper
- 10 ounces canned tuna, drained and flaked
- 1-pint cherry tomatoes, halved
- ½ cup pepperoncini, sliced
- ⅓ cup parsley, chopped
- 1 tablespoon olive oil
- ¼ cup capers, drained
- Juice of ½ lemon

Nutritions: Calories: 253, Fat: 11.5, Fiber: 3.4, Carbs: 16.5, Protein: 23.2

41. Garlic Rice

Preparation:
5 Minutes

Cooking:
3 Minutes

Servings:
4

Directions

1. Heat the oil in a large frying pan over a medium heat. When the oil is hot, add the garlic and ground pork. Boil and stir until garlic is golden brown.
2. Stir in cooked white rice and season with garlic salt and pepper. Bake and stir until the mixture is hot and well mixed for about 3 minutes.

Ingredients

- 2 tablespoons vegetable oil
- 1 ½ tablespoons chopped garlic
- 2 tablespoons ground pork
- 4 cups cooked white rice
- 1 1/2 teaspoons of garlic salt
- Ground black pepper to taste

Nutritions: *Calories: 293, Fat: 9g, Carbohydrates: 45.9g, Protein: 5.9g, Cholesterol: 6mg, Sodium: 686mg*

42. Carrot Rice

Preparation:
5 Minutes

Cooking:
25 Minutes

Servings:
6

Directions

1. Bring the water to a boil in a medium-sized saucepan over medium heat. Place in the bouillon cube and let it dissolve.
2. Stir in the carrots and rice and bring to a boil again.
3. Lower the heat, cover, and simmer for 20 minutes.
4. Remove from heat and leave under cover for 5 minutes.

Ingredients

- 2 cups of water
- 1 cube chicken broth
- 1 grated carrot
- 1 cup uncooked long-grain rice

Nutritions: Calories 125, Fat 0.3g, Carbohydrates 27.1g, Protein 2.7g, Cholesterol <1mg, Sodium 199mg

43. Seafood and Veggie Pasta

Preparation:
10 Minutes

Cooking:
20 Minutes

Servings:
4

Ingredients

- ¼ tsp pepper
- ¼ tsp salt
- 1 lb. raw shelled shrimp
- 1 lemon, cut into wedges
- 1 tbsp butter
- 1 tbsp olive oil
- 2 5-oz cans chopped clams, drained (reserve 2 tbsp clam juice)
- 2 tbsp dry white wine
- 4 cloves garlic, minced
- 4 cups zucchini, spiraled (use a veggie spiralizer)
- 4 tbsp Parmesan cheese
- Chopped fresh parsley to garnish

Directions

1. Prepare the zucchini and spiralize with a veggie spiralizer. Arrange 1 cup of zucchini noodles per bowl for a total of 4 bowls.
2. On medium fire, place a large nonstick saucepan and heat oil and butter.
3. For a minute, sauté garlic. Add shrimp and cook for 3 minutes until opaque or cooked.
4. Add white wine, reserved clam juice, and clams. Bring to a simmer and continue simmering for 2 minutes or until half of the liquid has evaporated. Stir constantly.
5. Season with pepper and salt. And if needed add more to taste.
6. Remove from fire and evenly distribute seafood sauce to 4 bowls.
7. Top with a tablespoonful of Parmesan cheese per bowl, serve and enjoy.

Nutritions: *Calories: 324.9, Carbohydrates: 12g, Protein: 43.8g, Fat: 11.3g*

44. Alethea's Lemony Asparagus Pasta

Preparation:
10 Minutes

Cooking:
20 Minutes

Servings:
6

Ingredients

- 1-pound spaghetti, linguini, or angel hair pasta
- 2 crusty bread slices
- ½ cup plus 1 tablespoon avocado oil, divided
- 3 cups chopped asparagus (1½-inch pieces)
- ½ cup vegan "chicken" broth or vegetable broth, divided
- 6 tablespoons freshly squeezed lemon juice
- 8 garlic cloves, minced or pressed
- 3 tablespoons finely chopped fresh curly parsley
- 1 tablespoon grated lemon zest
- 1½ teaspoons sea salt

Directions

1. Bring a large pot of water to a boil over high heat and cook the pasta until al dente according to the instructions on the package.
2. Meanwhile, in a medium skillet, crumble the bread into coarse crumbs. Add 1 tablespoon of oil to the pan and stir well to combine over medium heat. Cook for about 5 minutes, stirring often until the crumbs are golden brown. Remove from the skillet and set aside.
3. Add the chopped asparagus and ¼ cup of broth in the skillet and cook over medium-high heat until the asparagus is bright green and crisp-tender, about 5 minutes. Transfer the asparagus to a very large bowl.
4. Add the remaining ½ cup of oil, remaining ¼ cup of broth, lemon juice, garlic, parsley, zest, and salt to the asparagus bowl and stir well.
5. When the noodles are done, drain well, and add them to the bowl. Gently toss with the asparagus mixture. Just before serving, stir in the toasted breadcrumbs. Store leftovers in an airtight container in the refrigerator for up to 2 days.

Nutritions: Calories: 526, Total Fat: 23g, Saturated Fat: 3g, Protein: 13g, Carbohydrates: 68g, Fiber: 10g, Sodium: 1422mg, Iron: 6mg

45. Mushroom and Vegetable Penne Pasta

Preparation:
5 Minutes

Cooking:
8 Minutes

Servings:
4

Directions

1. Heat the oil
2. Sauté and stir-fry carrot and garlic for 3-4 minutes
3. Add remaining ingredients and pour in 2 cups water
4. Cook on high pressure for 4 minutes
5. Quick release the pressure
6. Serve and enjoy!

Ingredients

- 6 ounces penne pasta
- 6 ounces shiitake mushrooms, chopped
- 1 small carrot, cut into strips
- 4 ounces baby spinach, finely chopped
- 1 teaspoon ginger, grounded
- 3 tablespoons oil
- 2 tablespoons soy sauce
- 6 ounces zucchini, cut into strips
- 6 ounces leek, finely chopped
- ½ teaspoon salt
- 2 garlic cloves, crushed
- 2 cups of water

Nutritions: *Calories: 429, Fat: 8g, Carbohydrates: 64g, Protein: 25g*

MEDITERRANEAN DIET COOKBOOK *for beginners*

46. Broccoli and Orecchiette Pasta with Feta

Preparation:
10 Minutes

Cooking:
14 Minutes

Servings:
4

Ingredients

- 1 pack (9 ounces) orecchiette
- 1 tablespoon feta, grated
- 16 ounces broccoli, roughly chopped
- 2 garlic cloves
- 1 teaspoon salt
- ¼ teaspoon black pepper
- 3 tablespoons olive oil

Directions

1. Add broccoli and orecchiette into your instant pot
2. Cover with water and close the lid
3. Cook on high pressure for 10 minutes
4. Quick release the pressure
5. Drain the broccoli and orecchiette
6. Set them aside and then heat the oil on sauté mode
7. Stir-fry garlic for 2 minutes
8. Stir in orecchiette, broccoli, salt, and pepper
9. Cook for 2 minutes more
10. Once cooked, then press cancel and stir in grated feta
11. Serve and enjoy!

Nutritions: Calories: 350, Fat: 20g, Carbohydrates: 32g, Protein: 15g

47. Fiber Packed Chicken Rice

Preparation:
10 Minutes

Cooking:
16 Minutes

Servings:
6

Directions

1. Warm oil into the pot, then put garlic and onion and sauté for 2 minutes.
2. Add chicken and cook for 2 minutes. Add remaining ingredients and stir well.
3. Cook on high for 12 minutes. Stir well and serve.

Ingredients

- 1 lb. chicken breast, skinless, boneless, and cut into chunks
- 14.5 oz canned cannellini beans
- 4 cups chicken broth
- 2 cups wild rice
- 1 tbsp Italian seasoning
- 1 small onion, chopped
- 1 tbsp garlic, chopped
- 1 tbsp olive oil
- Pepper
- Salt

Nutritions: *Calories: 399, Fat: 6.4g, Carbohydrates: 53.4g, Sugar: 3g, Protein: 31.6g, Cholesterol: 50mg*

48. Tasty Greek Rice

Preparation: 10 Minutes

Cooking: 10 Minutes

Servings: 6

Directions

1. Put rice in a pot with olive oil and cook for 5 minutes.
2. Add remaining ingredients except for red peppers and olives and stir well—cook on high for 5 minutes.
3. Add red peppers and olives and stir well. Serve and enjoy.

Ingredients

- 1 3/4 cup brown rice, rinsed and drained
- 3/4 cup roasted red peppers, chopped
- 1 cup olives, chopped
- 1 tsp dried oregano
- 1 tsp Greek seasoning
- 1 3/4 cup vegetable broth
- 2 tbsp olive oil
- Salt

Nutritions: Calories: 285, Fat: 9.1g, Carbohydrates: 45.7g, Sugar: 1.2g, Protein: 6g, Cholesterol: 0mg

CHAPTER 11:
Seafood and Fish Recipes

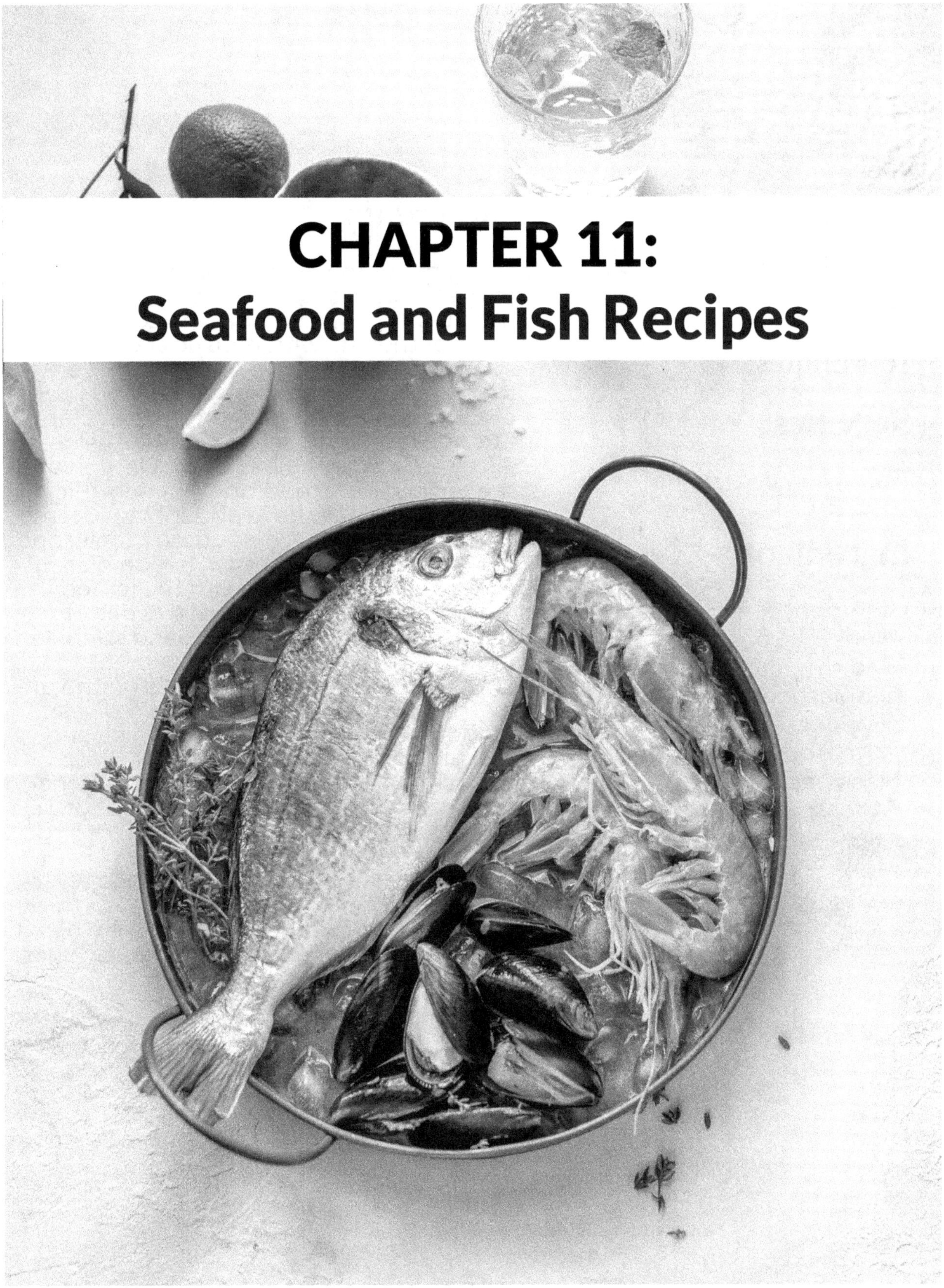

49. Grilled Fish on Lemons

Preparation:
10 Minutes

Cooking:
10 Minutes

Servings:
4

Ingredients

- 4 (4-ounce) fish fillets
- Nonstick cooking spray
- 3 to 4 medium lemons
- 1 tablespoon extra-virgin olive oil
- ¼ teaspoon freshly ground black pepper
- ¼ teaspoon kosher or sea salt

Directions

1. Using paper towels, pat the fillets dry and let stand at room temperature for 10 minutes. Meanwhile, coat the cold cooking grate of the grill with nonstick cooking spray, and preheat the grill to 400°F, or medium-high heat. Or preheat a grill pan over medium-high heat on the stovetop.
2. Cut one lemon in half and set half aside. Slice the remaining half of that lemon and the remaining lemons into ¼-inch-thick slices. You should have about 12 to 16 lemon slices. In a small bowl, squeeze 1 tablespoon of juice out of the reserved lemon half.
3. Add the oil to the bowl with the lemon juice and mix well. Brush both sides of the fish with the oil mixture, and sprinkle evenly with pepper and salt.
4. Carefully place the lemon slices on the grill (or the grill pan), arranging 3 to 4 slices together in the shape of a fish fillet, and repeat with the remaining slices. Place the fish fillets directly on top of the lemon slices, and grill with the lid closed. If you're grilling on the stovetop, cover with a large pot lid or aluminum foil. Turn the fish halfway through the cooking time only if the fillets are more than half an inch thick. The fish is done and ready to serve when it just begins to separate into flakes (chunks) when pressed gently with a fork.

Nutritions: Calories: 147, Fat: 5g, Fiber: 1g, Protein: 22g

50. Vinegar Honeyed Salmon

Preparation:
10 Minutes

Cooking:
5 Minutes

Servings:
4

Directions

1. In a mixing bowl, add honey and vinegar. Mix together well.
2. Season fish fillets with the black pepper (ground) and sea salt; brush with honey glaze. Take a medium saucepan or skillet, add oil. Heat over medium heat. Add salmon fillets and stir-cook until medium-rare in the center and lightly browned for 3-4 minutes per side. Serve warm.

Ingredients

- 4 (8-ounce) salmon fillets
- 1/2 cup balsamic vinegar
- 1 tablespoon honey
- Black pepper (ground) and sea salt, to taste
- 1 tablespoon olive oil

Nutritions: *Calories: 481, Fat: 16g, Carbohydrates: 24g, Fiber: 1.5g*

51. Orange Fish Meal

Preparation:
10 Minutes

Preparation:
5 Minutes

Servings:
4

Directions

1. Take a baking dish of 9-inch; add olive oil, orange juice, and salt. Mix well. Add fish fillets and coat well. Add onions over fish fillets. Cover with plastic wrap. Microwave for 3 minutes until fish is cooked well and easy to flake. Serve warm with sliced avocado on top.

Ingredients

- ¼ teaspoon kosher or sea salt
- 1 tablespoon extra-virgin olive oil
- 1 tablespoon orange juice
- 4 (4-ounce) tilapia fillets, with or without skin
- ¼ cup chopped red onion
- 1 avocado, pitted, skinned, and sliced

Nutritions: Calories: 231, Fat: 9g, Carbohydrates: 8g, Fiber: 2.5g

52. Shrimp Zoodles

Preparation:
10 Minutes

Preparation:
5 Minutes

Servings:
2

Ingredients

- 2 tablespoons chopped parsley
- 2 teaspoons minced garlic
- 1 teaspoon salt
- ½ teaspoon black pepper
- 2 medium zucchinis, spiralized
- 3/4 pounds medium shrimp, peeled & deveined
- 1 tablespoon olive oil
- 1 lemon, juiced and zested

Directions

1. Take a medium saucepan or skillet, add oil, lemon juice, and lemon zest. Heat over a medium heat. Add shrimps and stir-cook 1 minute per side. Add garlic and red pepper flakes; cook for 1 more minute.
2. Add zoodles and stir gently; cook for 3 minutes until cooked to satisfaction. Season with salt and black pepper and serve warm with parsley on top.

Nutritions: *Calories: 329, Fat: 12g, Carbohydrates: 11g, Fiber: 3g*

53. Tuna Nutty Salad

Preparation:
10 Minutes

Cooking:
0 Minutes

Servings:
4

Directions

1. In a large salad bowl, add tuna, shallot, chives, tarragon, and celery. Combine to mix well with each other. In a mixing bowl, add mayonnaise, mustard, salt, and black pepper. Combine to mix well with each other. Add mayonnaise mixture to a salad bowl; toss well to combine. Add pine nuts and toss again. Serve fresh.

Ingredients

- 1 tablespoon chopped tarragon
- 1 stalk celery, trimmed and finely diced
- 1 medium shallot, diced
- 3 tablespoons chopped chives
- 1 (5-ounce) can tuna (covered in olive oil) drained and flaked
- 1 teaspoon Dijon mustard
- 2-3 tablespoons mayonnaise
- 1/4 teaspoon salt
- 1/8 teaspoon pepper
- 1/4 cup pine nuts, toasted

Nutritions: Calories: 236, Fat: 14g, Carbohydrates: 4g, Fiber: 1g

54. Salmon Skillet Supper

Preparation:
15 Minutes

Cooking:
15 Minutes

Servings:
4

Ingredients

- 1 tablespoon extra-virgin olive oil
- 2 garlic cloves minced
- 1 teaspoon smoked paprika
- 1-pint grape or cherry tomatoes, quartered
- 1 (12-ounce) jar roasted red peppers
- 1 tablespoon water
- ¼ teaspoon freshly ground black pepper
- ¼ teaspoon kosher or sea salt
- 1-pound salmon fillets, skin removed, cut into 8 pieces
- 1 tablespoon freshly squeezed lemon juice (from ½ medium lemon)

Directions

1. In a large skillet over medium heat, heat the oil. Add the garlic and smoked paprika and cook for 1 minute, stirring often. Add the tomatoes, roasted peppers, water, black pepper, and salt. Turn up the heat to medium-high, bring to a simmer, and cook for 3 minutes, stirring occasionally and smashing the tomatoes with a wooden spoon toward the end of the cooking time.
2. Add the salmon to the skillet, and spoon some of the sauce over the top. Cover and cook for 10 to 12 minutes, or until the salmon is cooked through (145°F using a meat thermometer) and just starts to flake.
3. Remove the skillet from the heat, and drizzle lemon juice over the top of the fish. Stir the sauce, then break up the salmon into chunks with a fork. You can serve it straight from the skillet.

Nutritions: *Calories: 289, Total Fat: 13g, Fiber: 2g, Protein: 31g*

55. Weeknight Sheet Pan Fish Dinner

Preparation:
10 Minutes

Cooking:
10 Minutes

Servings:
4

Ingredients

- Nonstick cooking spray
- 2 tablespoons extra-virgin olive oil
- 1 tablespoon balsamic vinegar
- 4 (4-ounce) fish fillets (½ inch thick)
- 2½ cups green beans
- 1-pint cherry or grape tomatoes

Directions

1. Preheat the oven to 400°F. Coat two large, rimmed baking sheets with nonstick cooking spray. In a small bowl, whisk together the oil and vinegar. Set aside. Place two pieces of fish on each baking sheet.
2. In a large bowl, combine the beans and tomatoes. Pour in the oil and vinegar and toss gently to coat. Pour half of the green bean mixture over the fish on one baking sheet, and the remaining half over the fish on the other. Turn the fish over and rub it in the oil mixture to coat. Spread the vegetables evenly on the baking sheets so hot air can circulate around them.
3. Bake for 5 to 8 minutes, until the fish is just opaque and not translucent. The fish is done and ready to serve when it just begins to separate into flakes (chunks) when pressed gently with a fork.

Nutritions: Calories: 193, Fat: 8g, Fiber: 3g, Protein: 23g

56. Crispy Polenta Fish Sticks

Preparation:
15 Minutes

Cooking:
10 Minutes

Servings:
4

Ingredients

- 2 large eggs, lightly beaten
- 1 tablespoon 2% milk
- 1-pound skinned fish fillets sliced into 20 (1-inchwide) strips
- ½ cup yellow cornmeal
- ½ cup whole-wheat panko breadcrumbs
- ¼ teaspoon smoked paprika
- ¼ teaspoon kosher or sea salt
- ¼ teaspoon freshly ground black pepper
- Nonstick cooking spray

Directions

1. Place a large, rimmed baking sheet in the oven. Preheat the oven to 400°F with the pan inside. In a large bowl, mix the eggs and milk. Using a fork, add the fish strips to the egg mixture and stir gently to coat.
2. Put the cornmeal, breadcrumbs, smoked paprika, salt, and pepper in a quart-size zip-top plastic bag. Using a fork or tongs, transfer the fish to the bag, letting the excess egg drip off into the bowl before transferring. Seal the bag and shake gently to completely coat each fish stick.
3. With oven mitts, carefully remove the hot baking sheet from the oven and spray it with nonstick cooking spray. Using a fork or tongs, remove the fish sticks from the bag and arrange them on the hot baking sheet, with space between them so the hot air can circulate and crisp them up. Bake for 5 to 8 minutes, until gentle pressure with a fork causes the fish to flake, then serve.

Nutritions: *Calories: 256, Fat: 6g, Fiber: 2g, Protein: 29g*

57. Tuscan Tuna and Zucchini Burgers

Preparation:
10 Minutes

Cooking:
10 Minutes

Servings:
4

Ingredients

- 3 slices whole-wheat sandwich bread, toasted
- 2 (5-ounce) cans tuna in olive oil, drained
- 1 cup shredded zucchini
- 1 large egg, lightly beaten
- ¼ cup diced red bell pepper
- 1 tablespoon dried oregano
- 1 teaspoon lemon zest
- ¼ teaspoon freshly ground black pepper
- ¼ teaspoon kosher or sea salt
- 1 tablespoon extra-virgin olive oil
- Salad greens or 4 whole-wheat rolls, for serving (optional)

Directions

1. Crumble the toast into breadcrumbs using your fingers (or use a knife to cut into ¼-inch cubes) until you have 1 cup of loosely packed crumbs. Pour the crumbs into a large bowl. Add the tuna, zucchini, egg, bell pepper, oregano, lemon zest, black pepper, and salt. Mix well with a fork. With your hands, form the mixture into four (½-cup-size) patties. Place on a plate and press each patty flat to about ¾-inch thick.
2. In a large skillet over medium-high heat, heat the oil until it's very hot, about 2 minutes. Add the patties to the hot oil, then turn the heat down to medium. Cook the patties for 5 minutes, flip with a spatula, and cook for an additional 5 minutes. Enjoy as is or serve with salad greens or whole-wheat rolls.

Nutritions: Calories: 191, Fat: 10g, Fiber: 2g, Protein: 15g

58. Asparagus Trout Meal

Preparation:
10 Minutes

Cooking:
20 Minutes

Servings:
4

Ingredients

- 2 pounds trout fillets
- 1-pound asparagus
- Salt and ground white pepper, to taste
- 1 tablespoon olive oil
- 1 garlic clove, finely minced
- 1 scallion, thinly sliced (green and white part)
- 4 medium golden potatoes, thinly sliced
- 2 Roma tomatoes, chopped
- 8 pitted kalamata olives, chopped
- 1 large carrot, thinly sliced
- 2 tablespoons dried parsley
- ¼ cup ground cumin
- 2 tablespoons paprika
- 1 tablespoon vegetable bouillon seasoning
- ½ cup dry white wine

Directions

1. In a mixing bowl, add fish fillets, white pepper, and salt. Combine to mix well with each other. Take a medium saucepan or skillet and add oil. Heat over a medium heat. Add asparagus, potatoes, garlic, and white part scallion, and stir-cook until the mixture becomes softened for 4-5 minutes. Add tomatoes, carrot, and olives; stir-cook for 6-7 minutes until tender. Add cumin, paprika, parsley, bouillon seasoning, and salt. Stir the mixture well.
2. Mix in white wine and fish fillets. Over a low heat, cover and simmer the mixture for about 6 minutes until fish is easy to flake, stirring in between. Serve warm with green scallions on top.

Nutritions: *Calories: 303, Fat: 17g, Carbohydrates: 37g, Fiber: 6g*

59. Kale Olive Tuna

Preparation:
10 Minutes

Cooking:
15 Minutes

Servings:
6

Ingredients

- 1 cup chopped onion
- 3 garlic cloves, minced
- 1 (2.25-ounce) can sliced olives, drained
- 1-pound kale, chopped
- 3 tablespoons extra-virgin olive oil
- ¼ cup capers
- ¼ teaspoon crushed red pepper
- 2 teaspoons sugar
- 1 (15-ounce) can cannellini beans or great northern beans, drained
- 2 (6-ounce) cans tuna in olive oil, un-drained
- ¼ teaspoon black pepper
- ¼ teaspoon kosher or sea salt

Directions

1. Cook the kale in boiling water for 2 minutes; drain and set aside. Take a medium-large cooking pot or stockpot andheat the oil over z medium heat. Add onion and stir-cook until translucent and softened. Add garlic and stir-cook for 1 minute.
2. Add olives, capers, and red pepper, and stir-cook for 1 minute. Mix in cooked kale and sugar. Over a low heat, cover and simmer the mixture for about 8-10 minutes, stirring in between. Add tuna, beans, pepper, and salt. Stir well and serve warm.

Nutritions: Calories: 242, Fat: 11g, Carbohydrates: 24g, Fiber: 7g

60. Tangy Rosemary Shrimps

Preparation:
10 Minutes

Cooking:
10 Minutes

Servings:
6

Ingredients

- 1 large orange, zested and peeled
- 3 garlic cloves, minced
- 1 ½ pounds raw shrimp, shells, and tails removed
- 3 tablespoons olive oil
- 1 tablespoon chopped thyme
- 1 tablespoon chopped rosemary
- ¼ teaspoon black pepper
- ¼ teaspoon kosher or sea salt

Directions

1. Take a zip-top plastic bag, add orange zest, shrimps, 2 tablespoons olive oil, garlic, thyme, rosemary, salt, and black pepper. Shake well and set aside to marinate for 5 minutes.
2. Take a medium saucepan or skillet, add 1 tablespoon olive oil. Heat over medium heat. Add shrimps and stir-cook for 2-3 minutes per side until totally pink and opaque. Slice the orange into bite-sized wedges and add in a serving plate. Add shrimp and combine well. Serve fresh.

Nutritions: *Calories: 187, Fat: 7g, Carbohydrates: 6g, Fiber: 0.5g*

61. Asparagus Salmon

Preparation:
10 Minutes

Cooking:
15 Minutes

Servings:
2

Directions

1. Season salmon fillets with salt and black pepper. Take a medium saucepan or skillet, add oil. Heat over medium heat. Add salmon fillets and stir-cook until evenly seared and cooked well for 4-5 minutes per side. Add asparagus and stir cook for 4-5 more minutes. Serve warm with hollandaise sauce on top.

Ingredients

- 8.8-ounce bunch asparagus
- 2 small salmon fillets
- 1 ½ teaspoon salt
- 1 teaspoon black pepper
- 1 tablespoon olive oil
- 1 cup hollandaise sauce, low-carb

Nutritions: Calories: 565, Fat: 7g, Carbohydrates: 8g, Fiber: 2.5g

62. Sicilian Kale and Tuna Bowl

Preparation:
15 Minutes

Cooking:
15 Minutes

Servings:
6

Ingredients

- 1-pound kale
- 3 tablespoons extra-virgin olive oil
- 1 cup chopped onion
- 3 garlic cloves, minced
- 1 (2.25-ounce) can sliced olives, drained
- ¼ cup capers
- ¼ teaspoon crushed red pepper
- 2 teaspoons sugar
- 2 (6-ounce) cans tuna in olive oil, undrained
- 1 (15-ounce) can cannellini beans or great northern beans
- ¼ teaspoon freshly ground black pepper
- ¼ teaspoon kosher or sea salt

Directions

1. Fill a large stockpot three-quarters full of water and bring to a boil. Add the kale and cook for 2 minutes. (This is to make the kale less bitter.) Drain the kale in a colander and set aside.
2. Set the empty pot back on the stove over medium heat and pour in the oil. Add the onion and cook for 4 minutes, stirring often. Add the garlic and cook for 1 minute, stirring often. Add the olives, capers, and crushed red pepper, and cook for 1 minute, stirring often. Add the partially cooked kale and sugar, stirring until the kale is completely coated with oil. Cover the pot and cook for 8 minutes.
3. Remove the kale from the heat, mix in the tuna, beans, pepper, and salt, and serve.

Nutritions: *Calories 265, Total Fat: 12g, Fiber: 7g, Protein: 16g*

63. Mediterranean Cod Stew

Preparation:
10 Minutes

Cooking:
20 Minutes

Servings:
6

Ingredients

- 2 tablespoons extra-virgin olive oil
- 2 cups chopped onion
- 2 garlic cloves, minced
- ¾ teaspoon smoked paprika
- 1 (14.5-ounce) can diced tomatoes, undrained
- 1 (12-ounce) jar roasted red peppers
- 1 cup sliced olives, green or black
- ⅓ cup dry red wine
- ¼ teaspoon freshly ground black pepper
- ¼ teaspoon kosher or sea salt
- 1½ pounds cod fillets, cut into 1-inch pieces
- 3 cups sliced mushrooms

Directions

1. In a large stockpot over medium heat, heat the oil. Add the onion and cook for 4 minutes, stirring occasionally. Add the garlic and smoked paprika and cook for 1 minute, stirring often.
2. Mix in the tomatoes with their juices, roasted peppers, olives, wine, pepper, and salt, and turn the heat up to medium-high. Bring to a boil. Add the cod and mushrooms and reduce the heat to medium.
3. Cover and cook for about 10 minutes, stirring a few times, until the cod is cooked through and flakes easily. Serve.

Nutritions: Calories: 220, Fat: 8g, Fiber: 3g, Protein: 28g

CHAPTER 12:
Poultry Recipes

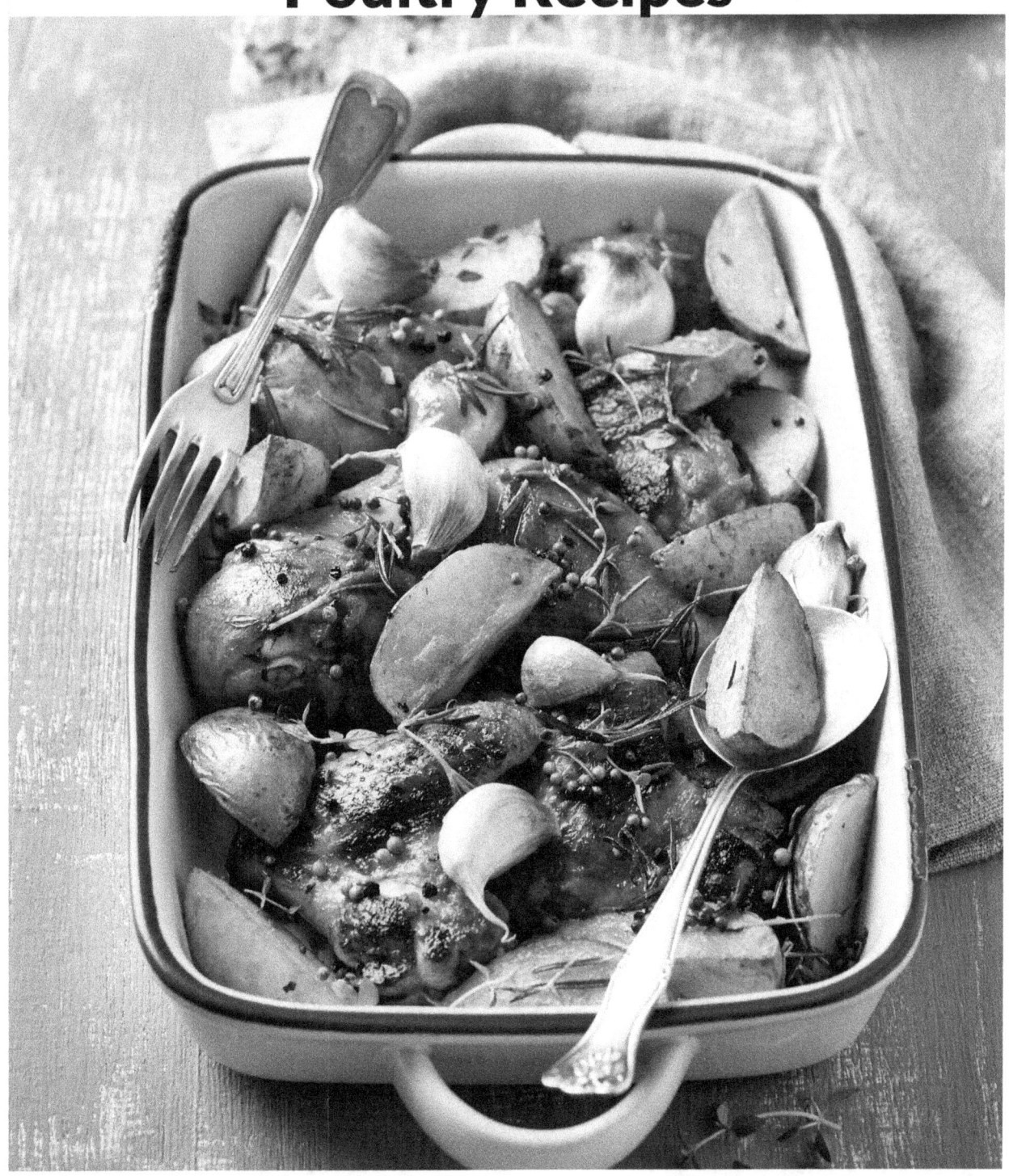

64. Cacciatore Black Olive Chicken

Preparation:
10 Minutes

Cooking:
15 Minutes

Servings:
4-6

Ingredients

- 6–8 bone-in chicken drumsticks or mixed drumsticks and thighs
- 1 cup chicken stock
- 1 bay leaf
- ½ cup black olives, pitted
- 1 medium yellow onion, roughly chopped
- 1 teaspoon dried oregano
- 1 teaspoon garlic powder
- 1 (28-ounce) can stewed tomato puree

Directions

1. Open the top lid of your Instant Pot.
2. Add the stock, bay leaf, and salt; stir to combine with a wooden spatula.
3. Add the chicken, tomato puree, onion, garlic powder, and oregano; stir again.
4. Close the lid and make sure that the valve is sealed properly.
5. Press 'Manual' and set the timer to 15 minutes.
6. The Instant Pot will start building pressure; allow the mixture to cook for the set time.
7. When the timer reads zero, press 'NPR' for natural pressure release. It will take 8–10 minutes to release the pressure.
8. Open the lid and remove the bay leaf.
9. Serve warm with the black olives on top.

Nutritions: Calories: 309, Fat: 16.5g, Carbs: 9g, Protein: 30.5g, Sodium: 833mg

65. Mustard Green Chicken

Preparation:
10 Minutes

Cooking:
15 Minutes

Servings:
4

Ingredients

- 1 bunch mustard greens, washed and chopped
- Juice of 1 lemon
- ⅓ cup extra-virgin olive oil
- 4–5 boneless, skinless chicken thighs
- 3 cloves garlic, minced
- 1 cup white wine
- 1 teaspoon Dijon mustard
- 1 teaspoon honey
- ½ cup cherry tomatoes
- ½ cup green olives, pitted
- Salt and pepper to taste

Directions

1. Open the top lid of your Instant Pot.
2. Add the mustard greens and then add the chicken thighs on top; season to taste with salt and pepper.
3. Top with the garlic, tomatoes, olives, mustard, and honey followed by the lemon juice, olive oil, and wine.
4. Close the lid and make sure that the valve is sealed properly.
5. Press 'Manual' and set the timer to 15 minutes.
6. The Instant Pot will start building pressure; allow the mixture to cook for the set time.
7. When the timer reads zero, press 'QPR' for quick pressure release.
8. Open the lid and take out the prepared recipe.
9. Serve warm.

Nutritions: *Calories: 314, Fat: 19g, Carbs: 14.5g, Protein: 17g, Sodium: 745mg*

66. Chickpea Spiced Chicken

Preparation:
10 Minutes

Cooking:
15 Minutes

Servings:
4

Ingredients

- 2 red peppers, cut into chunks
- 1 large onion
- 1 (15-ounce) can chickpeas
- 4 cloves garlic
- 2 Roma tomatoes, cut into chunks
- 1 tablespoon olive oil
- 1–2 pounds boneless chicken thighs, trimmed and cut into large chunks
- 1 teaspoon cumin
- ½ teaspoon coriander powder
- 1 teaspoon salt
- ½ teaspoon pepper
- 1 teaspoon dried parsley
- ½ teaspoon red pepper flakes
- 1 cup tomato sauce

Directions

1. Open the top lid of your Instant Pot and press SAUTÉ.
2. Add the olive oil to the pot and heat it.
3. Add the onions and garlic and stircook for 4–5 minutes until soft and translucent.
4. Add chicken chunks; stir-cook for 4–5 minutes on each side to evenly brown.
5. Add the remaining ingredients and stir gently.
6. Close the lid and make sure that the valve is sealed properly.
7. Press 'Manual' and set the timer to 10 minutes.
8. The Instant Pot will start building pressure; allow the mixture to cook for the set time.
9. When the timer reads zero, press 'QPR' for quick pressure release.
10. Open the lid and take out the prepared recipe.
11. Serve warm with grilled pita (optional).

Nutritions: Calories: 371, Fat: 15g, Carbs: 26.5g, Protein: 33g, Sodium: 1279mg

67. Vegetable Rice Chicken

Preparation:
10 Minutes

Cooking:
4 Minutes

Servings:
4

Ingredients

- 1 medium red onion, diced
- 4 cloves garlic, minced
- 2 tablespoons olive oil
- 3 chicken breasts, diced
- 3 tablespoons lemon juice
- 1½ cups chicken broth
- 1 each red and yellow bell pepper, chopped
- 1 zucchini, sliced
- 1 cup dry white rice
- ¼ cup parsley, finely chopped
- 1 tablespoon oregano
- ½ teaspoon each salt and pepper
- ¼ cup feta cheese, crumbled (optional)

Directions

1. Open the top lid of your Instant Pot.
2. Add the olive oil, garlic, onions, chicken, lemon juice, oregano, salt, and pepper; stir to combine with a wooden spatula.
3. Add the broth and rice; stir again.
4. Close the lid and make sure that the valve is sealed properly.
5. Press 'Manual' and set the timer to 4 minutes.
6. The Instant Pot will start building pressure; allow the mixture to cook for the set time.
7. When the timer reads zero, press 'QPR' for quick pressure release.
8. Open the lid and stir in the bell peppers, zucchini, and parsley. Close the lid and allow to settle for 5–10 minutes.
9. Serve warm with feta cheese on top (optional).

Nutritions: *Calories: 293, Fat: 11g, Carbs: 33.5g, Protein: 16g, Sodium: 951mg*

68. Tender Chicken Quesadilla

Preparation:
10 Minutes

Cooking:
20 Minutes

Servings:
4

Ingredients

- 2 bread tortillas
- 1 teaspoon butter
- 2 teaspoons olive oil
- 1 teaspoon taco seasoning
- 6 oz chicken breast, skinless, boneless, sliced
- ⅓ cup Cheddar cheese, shredded
- 1 bell pepper, cut into wedges

Directions

1. Pour 1 teaspoon of olive oil into the skillet and add chicken.
2. Sprinkle the meat with Taco seasoning and mix up well.
3. Roast chicken for 10 minutes over a medium heat. Stir it from time to time.
4. Then transfer the cooked chicken to the plate.
5. Add remaining olive oil to the skillet.
6. Then add bell pepper and roast it for 5 minutes. Stir it all the time.
7. Mix together bell pepper with chicken.
8. Toss butter in the skillet and melt it.
9. Put 1 tortilla in the skillet.
10. Put Cheddar cheese on the tortilla and flatten it.
11. Then add the chicken-pepper mixture and cover it with the second tortilla.
12. Roast the quesadilla for 2 minutes on each side.
13. Cut the cooked meal on the halves and transfer to the serving plates.

Nutritions: Calories: 167, Fat: 8.2g, Fiber: 0.8g, Carbs: 16.4g, Protein: 24.2g

69. Light Caesar

Preparation:
10 Minutes

Cooking:
10 Minutes

Servings:
4

Ingredients

- 4 oz chicken fillet, chopped
- ¼ cup black olives, chopped
- 2 cups lettuce, chopped
- 1 tablespoon mayo sauce
- 1 teaspoon lemon juice
- ½ oz Parmesan cheese, shaved
- 1 teaspoon olive oil
- ½ teaspoon ground black pepper
- ½ teaspoon coconut oil

Directions

1. Sprinkle the chicken fillet with ground black pepper.
2. Heat up coconut oil and add chopped chicken fillet.
3. Roast it for 10 minutes or until it is cooked. Stir it from time to time.
4. Meanwhile, mix together black olives, lettuce, and Parmesan in the bowl.
5. Make mayo dressing: whisk together mayo sauce, olive oil, and lemon juice.
6. Add the cooked chicken to the salad and shake well.
7. Pour the mayo sauce dressing over the salad.

Nutritions: *Calories: 134, Fat: 13.3g, Fiber: 0g, Carbs: 2g, Protein: 9.4g*

70. Chicken Parm

Preparation:
10 Minutes

Cooking:
30 Minutes

Servings:
4

Ingredients

- 4 chicken steaks (4 oz each steak)
- ½ cup crushed tomatoes
- ¼ cup fresh cilantro
- 1 garlic clove, diced
- ½ cup of water
- 1 onion, diced
- 1 teaspoon olive oil
- 3 oz Parmesan, grated
- 3 tablespoon Panko breadcrumbs
- 2 eggs, beaten
- 1 teaspoon ground black pepper

Directions

1. Pour olive oil into the saucepan.
2. Add garlic and onion. Roast the vegetables for 3 minutes.
3. Then add fresh cilantro, crushed tomatoes, and water.
4. Simmer the mixture for 5 minutes.
5. Meanwhile, mix up together ground black pepper and eggs.
6. Dip the chicken steaks in the egg mixture.
7. Then coat them in Panko breadcrumbs and again in the egg mixture.
8. Coat the chicken steaks in grated Parmesan.
9. Place the prepared chicken steaks in the crushed tomato mixture.
10. Close the lid and cook chicken parm for 20 minutes. Flip the chicken steaks after 10 minutes of cooking.
11. Serve the chicken parm with crushed tomato sauce.

Nutritions: Calories: 354, Fat: 21.3g, Fiber: 2.1g, Carbs: 12g, Protein: 32.4g

71. Chicken Bolognese

Preparation:
7 Minutes

Cooking:
25 Minutes

Servings:
4

Ingredients

- 1 cup ground chicken
- 2 oz Parmesan, grated
- 1 tablespoon olive oil
- 2 tablespoons fresh parsley, chopped
- 1 teaspoon chili pepper
- 1 teaspoon paprika
- ½ teaspoon dried oregano
- ¼ teaspoon garlic, minced
- ½ teaspoon dried thyme
- ⅓ cup crushed tomatoes

Directions

1. Heat up olive oil in the skillet.
2. Add ground chicken and sprinkle it with chili pepper, paprika, dried oregano, dried thyme, and parsley. Mix up well.
3. Cook the chicken for 5 minutes and add crushed tomatoes. Mix up well.
4. Close the lid and simmer the chicken mixture for 10 minutes over a low heat.
5. Then add grated Parmesan and mix up.
6. Cook chicken bolognese for 5 minutes more over a medium heat.

Nutritions: *Calorie: 154, Fat: 9.3g, Fiber: 1.1g, Carbs: 3g, Protein: 15.4g*

72. Chicken Shawarma

Preparation:
10 Minutes

Cooking:
15 Minutes

Servings:
2-4

Ingredients

- 1–1½ pounds boneless skinless chicken thighs, cut into strips
- 1–1½ pounds boneless skinless chicken breasts, cut into strips
- ½ teaspoon turmeric
- 1 teaspoon ground cumin
- 1 teaspoon paprika
- ¼ teaspoon granulated garlic
- ⅛ teaspoon ground cinnamon
- ¼ teaspoon ground allspice
- ¼ teaspoon chili powder
- Salt and pepper to taste
- 1 cup chicken broth or stock

Directions

1. Combine the spices in a mixing bowl. Add the strips and coat well. Season to taste with salt and pepper.
2. Open the top lid of your Instant Pot.
3. Add the broth and chicken strips; stir to combine with a wooden spatula.
4. Close the lid and make sure that the valve is sealed properly.
5. Press 'Manual' and set the timer to 15 minutes.
6. The Instant Pot will start building pressure; allow the mixture to cook for the set time.
7. When the timer reads zero, press 'QPR' for quick pressure release.
8. Open the lid and take out the prepared recipe.
9. Serve warm with cooked veggies of your choice (optional).

Nutritions: Calories: 273, Fat: 9g, Carbs: 12.5g, Protein: 39.5g, Sodium: 1149mg

73. Caprese Chicken Dinner

Preparation:
10 Minutes

Cooking:
20 Minutes

Servings:
6

Ingredients

- ¼ cup maple syrup or honey
- ¼ cup chicken stock or water
- ¼ cup balsamic vinegar
- 1½ pounds boneless skinless chicken thighs, fat trimmed
- 8 slices mozzarella cheese
- 3 cups cherry tomatoes
- ½ cup basil leaves, torn

Directions

1. Open the top lid of your Instant Pot.
2. Add the stock, balsamic vinegar, and maple syrup; stir to combine with a wooden spatula.
3. Add the chicken thighs and combine them well.
4. Close the lid and make sure that the valve is sealed properly.
5. Press 'Manual' and set the timer to 10 minutes.
6. The Instant Pot will start building pressure; allow the mixture to cook for the set time.
7. When the timer reads zero, press 'QPR' for quick pressure release.
8. Open the lid, remove the chicken thighs, and place them on a baking sheet. Top each thigh with a cheese slice.
9. Press SAUTÉ; cook the sauce mixture for 4–5 minutes. Add the tomatoes and simmer for 1–2 minutes. Mix in the basil.
10. Add the baking sheet to a broiler and heat until the cheese melts. Serve warm with the sauce drizzled on top.

Nutritions: *Calories: 311, Fat: 13g, Carbs: 15g, Protein: 31g, Sodium: 364mg*

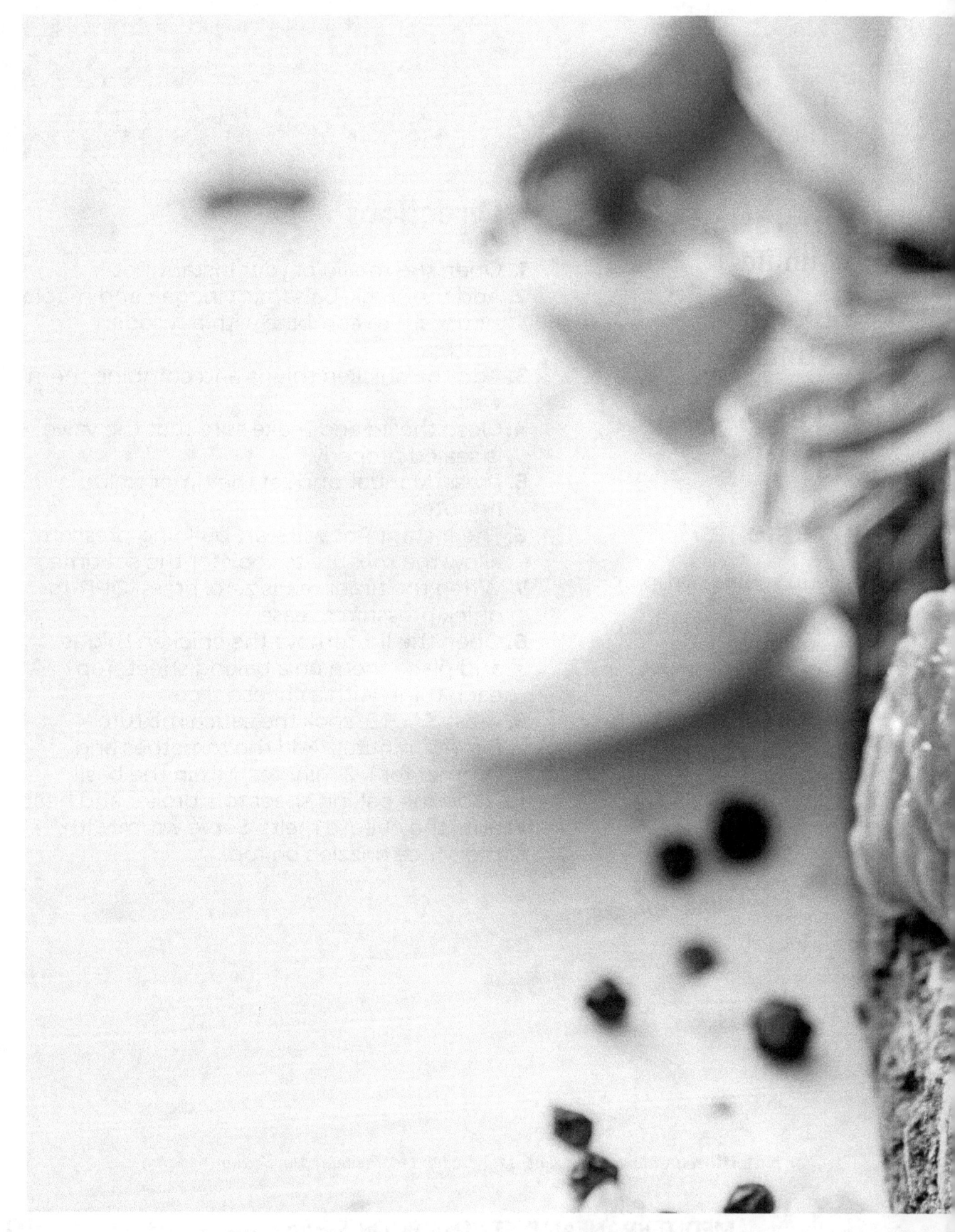

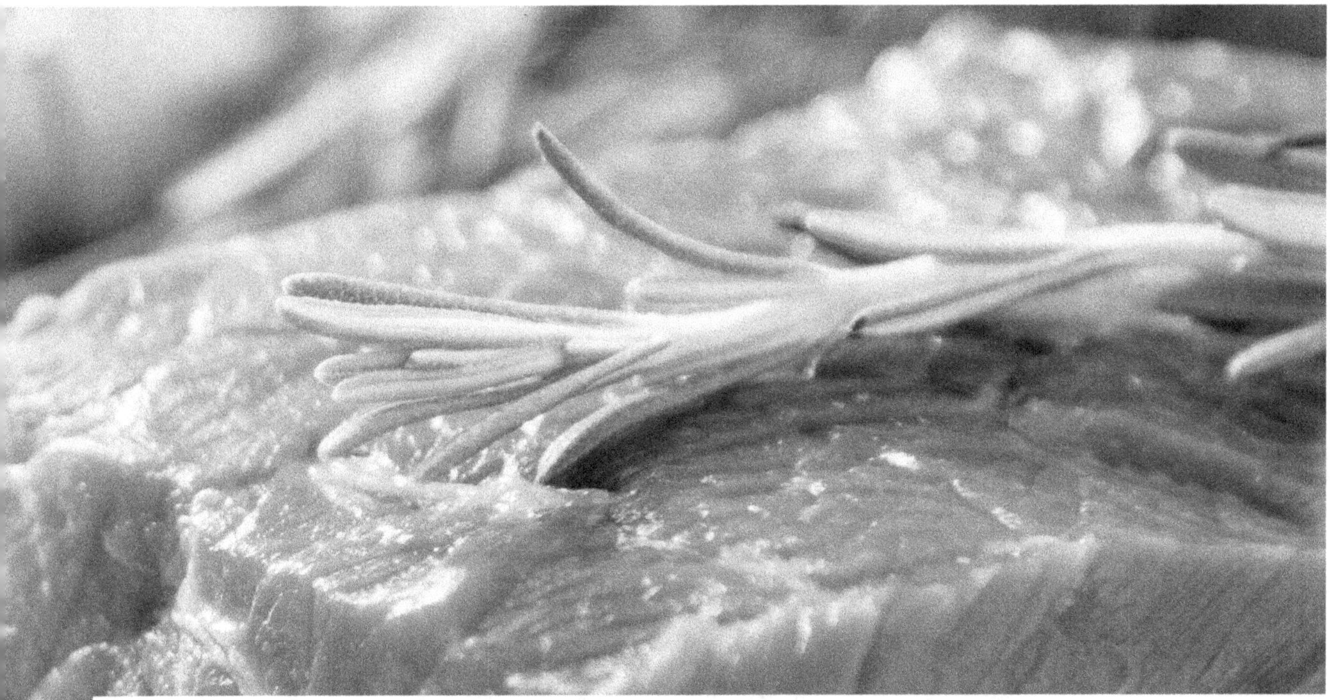

CHAPTER 13:
Meat and Eggs Recipes

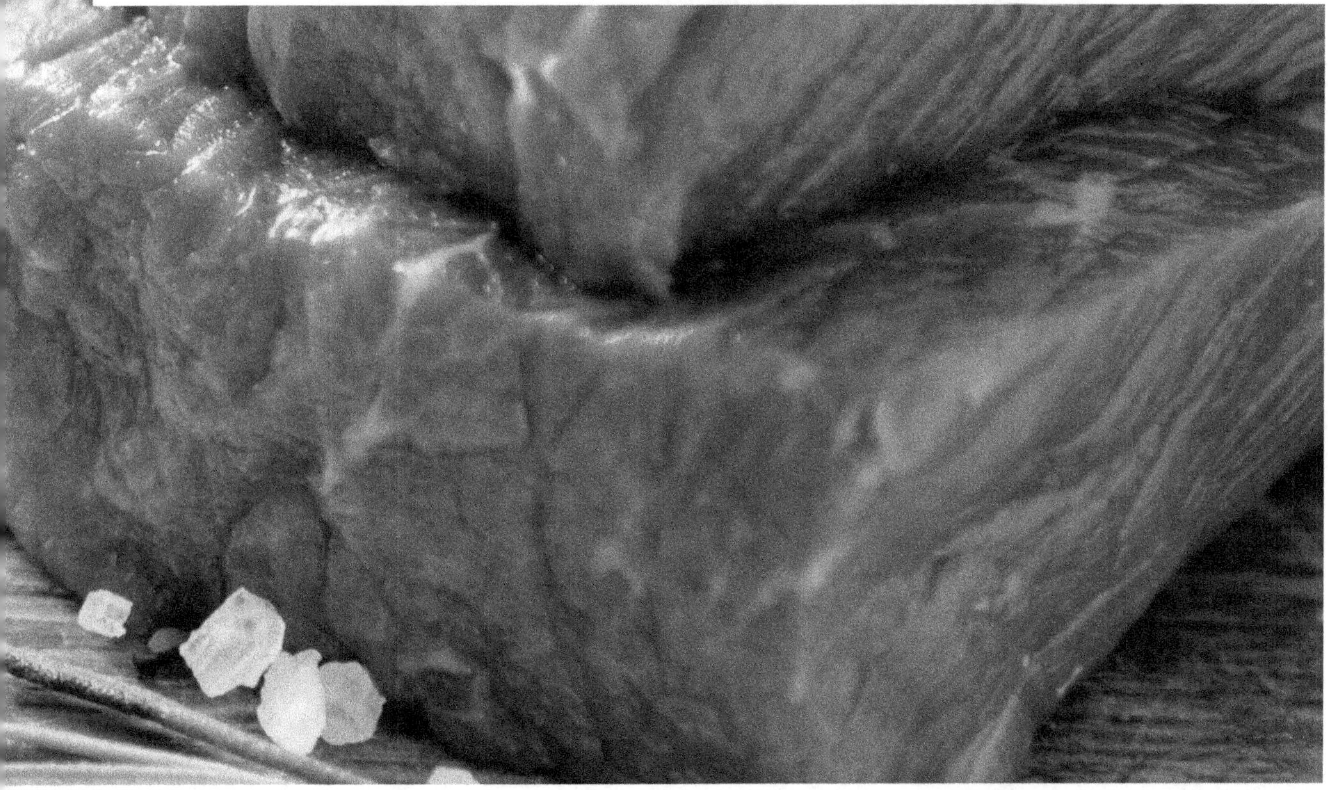

74. Mediterranean Grilled Pork Chops

Preparation:
1 Day

Cooking:
20 Minutes

Servings:
6

Ingredients

- 2 pork chops
- ¼ cup olive oil
- 2 yellow onions, sliced
- 2 garlic cloves, minced
- 2 teaspoons mustard
- 1 teaspoon sweet paprika
- Salt and black pepper to taste
- ½ teaspoon oregano, dried
- ½ teaspoon thyme, dried
- A pinch of cayenne pepper

Directions

1. In a small bowl, mix oil with garlic, mustard, paprika, black pepper, oregano, thyme, and cayenne and whisk well.
2. In a bowl, combine onions with meat and mustard mix, toss to coat, cover, and keep in the fridge for 1 day. Place meat on a preheated grill pan over medium-high heat, season with salt, and cook for 10 minutes on each side.
3. Meanwhile, heat a pan over a medium heat, add marinated onions, stir, and sauté for 4 minutes.
4. Divide pork chops on plates, add sautéed onions on top, and serve.

Nutritions: Calories: 234, Fat: 31g, Fiber: 15g, Carbs: 21g, Protein: 23g

75. Simple Pork Stir Fry

Preparation:
10 Minutes

Cooking:
15 Minutes

Servings:
4

Ingredients

- 4 ounces bacon, chopped
- 4 ounces snow peas
- 2 tablespoons butter
- 1-pound pork loin, cut into thin strips
- 2 cups mushrooms, sliced
- ¾ cup white wine
- ½ cup yellow onion, chopped
- 3 tablespoons sour cream
- Salt and white pepper to taste

Directions

1. Put snow peas in a saucepan, add water to cover, add a pinch of salt, bring to a boil over medium heat, cook until they are soft, drain and leave aside.
2. Heat a pan over a medium-high heat, add bacon, cook for a few minutes, drain grease, transfer to a bowl, and leave aside.
3. Heat a pan with 1 tablespoon butter over medium heat, add pork strips, salt, and pepper to taste, brown for a few minutes, and transfer to a plate as well.
4. Return pan to medium heat, add remaining butter, and melt it. Add onions and mushrooms, stir, and cook for 4 minutes.
5. Add wine, and simmer until it's reduced. Add cream, peas, pork, salt, and pepper to taste, stir, heat up, divide between plates, top with bacon, and serve.

Nutritions: *Calories: 343, Fat: 31g, Fiber: 15g, Carbs: 21g, Protein: 23g*

76. Pork and Lentil Soup

Preparation:
10 Minutes

Cooking:
1 Hour

Servings:
6

Ingredients

- 1 small yellow onion, chopped
- 1 tablespoon olive oil
- 1 and ½ teaspoons basil, chopped
- 1 and ½ teaspoons ginger, grated
- 3 garlic cloves, chopped
- Salt and black pepper to taste
- ½ teaspoon cumin, ground
- 1 carrot, chopped
- 1-pound pork chops, bone-in 3 ounces brown lentils, rinsed
- 3 cups chicken stock
- 2 tablespoons tomato paste
- 2 tablespoons lime juice
- 1 teaspoon red chili flakes, crushed

Directions

1. Heat a saucepan with the oil over medium heat, add garlic, onion, basil, ginger, salt, pepper, and cumin, stir well, and cook for 6 minutes.
2. Add carrots, stir, and cook for 5 more minutes. Add pork and brown for a few minutes.
3. Add lentils, tomato paste, and stock, stir, bring to a boil, cover pan and simmer for 50 minutes.
4. Transfer pork to a plate, discard bones, shred it and return to pan.
5. Add chili flakes and lime juice, stir, ladle into bowls, and serve.

Nutritions: Calories: 343, Fat: 31g, Fiber: 15g, Carbs: 21g, Protein: 23g

77. Simple Braised Pork

Preparation:
40 Minutes

Cooking:
1 Hour

Servings:
4

Ingredients

- 2 pounds pork loin roast, boneless and cubed
- 5 tablespoons butter
- Salt and black pepper to taste
- 2 cups chicken stock
- ½ cup dry white wine
- 2 garlic cloves, minced
- 1 teaspoon thyme, chopped
- 1 thyme sprig
- 1 bay leaf
- ½ yellow onion, chopped
- 2 tablespoons white flour
- ¾ pound pearl onions
- ½ pound red grapes

Directions

1. Heat a pan with 2 tablespoons butter over high heat, add pork loin, some salt, and pepper, stir, brown for 10 minutes, and transfer to a plate.
2. Add wine to the pan, bring to a boil over high heat and cook for 3 minutes.
3. Add stock, garlic, thyme spring, bay leaf, yellow onion and return meat to the pan, bring to a boil, cover, reduce heat to low, cook for 1 hour, strain liquid into another saucepan, and transfer pork to a plate.
4. Put pearl onions in a small saucepan, add water to cover, bring to a boil over medium-high heat, boil them for 5 minutes, drain, peel them, and leave aside for now.
5. In a bowl, mix 2 tablespoons butter with flour and stir well. Add ½ cup of strained cooking liquid and whisk well.
6. Pour this into cooking liquid, bring to a simmer over medium heat and cook for 5 minutes.
7. Add salt and pepper, chopped thyme, pork, and pearl onions, cover, and simmer for a few minutes.
8. Meanwhile, heat a pan with 1 tablespoon butter, add grapes, stir, and cook them for 1-2 minutes.
9. Divide pork meat on plates, drizzle the sauce all over, and serve with onions and grapes on the side.

Nutritions: *Calories: 343, Fat: 31g, Fiber: 15g, Carbs: 21g, Protein: 23g*

74. Mediterranean Grilled Pork Chops

Preparation:
1 Day

Cooking:
20 Minutes

Servings:
6

Ingredients

- 2 pork chops
- ¼ cup olive oil
- 2 yellow onions, sliced
- 2 garlic cloves, minced
- 2 teaspoons mustard
- 1 teaspoon sweet paprika
- Salt and black pepper to taste
- ½ teaspoon oregano, dried
- ½ teaspoon thyme, dried
- A pinch of cayenne pepper

Directions

1. In a small bowl, mix oil with garlic, mustard, paprika, black pepper, oregano, thyme, and cayenne and whisk well.
2. In a bowl, combine onions with meat and mustard mix, toss to coat, cover, and keep in the fridge for 1 day. Place meat on a preheated grill pan over medium-high heat, season with salt, and cook for 10 minutes on each side.
3. Meanwhile, heat a pan over a medium heat, add marinated onions, stir, and sauté for 4 minutes.
4. Divide pork chops on plates, add sautéed onions on top, and serve.

Nutritions: Calories: 320g, Fat: 31g, Fiber: 15g, Carbs: 21g, Protein: 23g

78. Caprese Poached Eggs

Preparation:
10 Minutes

Cooking:
10 Minutes

Servings:
2

Ingredients

- 1 tablespoon white vinegar (distilled)
- 4 eggs
- 1 tomato (sliced)
- 2 mozzarella cheese slices (1 ounce each)
- 4 teaspoon pesto
- 2 whole-wheat English muffins
- 2 teaspoons sea salt.

Directions

1. Place a large saucepan on your stove and fill it with 3 inches of water. Turn the heat to high so that the water can come to a boil. When the water starts boiling, add the tablespoon of vinegar to the saucepan and the salt, reduce the heat so that the water will maintain a gentle boil.
2. As the water simmers, Prepare your English muffins. Cut the muffins in half lengthwise. Place a slice of the mozzarella cheese on each muffin half then layer on a slice of tomato. Place the muffins on a cooking sheet and place them in your boiler. If you have a toaster oven you can use that instead of your broiler. Allow the muffins to toast up and the cheese to soften. This should take about 5 minutes.
3. As the muffins toast, crack an egg into a small bowl. Hold the bowl over the saucepan with the simmering water. Slowly pour the egg into the water, being careful not to break the yolk. Then repeat with the other three eggs. Once all eggs are in the water allow them to poach for about 3 minutes. The egg whites should be firm and fluffy.
4. As the eggs cook, place a few paper towels on a plate. Use a slotted spoon to transfer your cooked eggs to the plate to remove any excess water.
5. Remove your English muffin from the boiler or toaster oven.
6. Carefully transfer the muffin halves to a serving plate and place a poached egg on each half.
7. Take your pesto sauce and top each muffin with a tablespoon of the sauce. Serve and enjoy!

Nutritions: *Calories: 357, Carbs: 19g, Protein: 23g, Fat: 21.5g*

79. Sautéed Greens and Eggs

Preparation:
15 Minutes

Cooking:
15 Minutes

Servings:
4

Ingredients

- 1 tablespoon virgin olive oil
- 4 eggs
- 2 cups rainbow chard
- 1 cup spinach
- ½ cup arugula
- 2 garlic cloves (minced)
- ½ cup feta cheese
- ½ teaspoon sea salt
- ½ teaspoon black pepper

Directions

1. Place a large skillet on your stove with a tablespoon of virgin olive oil. Turn the heat on to medium-high.
2. As the skillet is heating, break your eggs into a medium-sized mixing bowl and use a fork to beat the eggs. Set to the side.
3. Your skillet should be nice and hot now. Add in your rainbow chard, spinach, and arugula, and allow the greens to sauté for about 5 minutes. Once the greens are nice and tender, add your minced garlic to the skillet and cook for two minutes.
4. Take your egg mixture and pour it into the skillet with your greens. Then sprinkle your feta cheese over top.
5. Cover the pan and then allow it to cook for 6 minutes.
6. Once the eggs have cooked thoroughly, uncover the skillet, and sprinkle the sea salt and black pepper over top.
7. Divide the mixture into four and serve.

Nutritions: Calories: 152, Protein: 9.2g, Fat: 11.9g, Carbs: 3g

80. Slow-Cooked Mediterranean Pork

Preparation:
20 Hours & 10 Minutes

Cooking:
8 Hours

Servings:
6

Ingredients

- 3 pounds pork shoulder - boneless
- ¼ cup olive oil
- 2 teaspoons oregano, dried
- ¼ cup lemon juice
- 2 teaspoons mustard
- 2 teaspoons mint, chopped
- 3 garlic cloves, minced
- 2 teaspoons pesto sauce
- Salt and black pepper to taste

Directions

1. In a bowl, mix olive oil with lemon juice, oregano, mint, mustard, garlic, pesto, salt, and pepper then whisk well.
2. Rub pork with marinade, cover, and keep in a cold place for 10 hours.
3. Flip pork shoulder and leave aside for 10 more hours.
4. Transfer to your slow cooker along with the marinade juices, cover, and cook on low for 8 hours.
5. Uncover, slice, divide between plates, and serve.

Nutritions: *Calories: 320, Fat: 31g, Fiber: 15g, Carbs: 21g, Protein: 23g*

81. Pork and Bean Stew

Preparation:
20 Minutes

Cooking:
20 Minutes

Servings:
4

Ingredients

- 2 pounds pork neck
- 1 tablespoon white flour
- 1 and ½ tablespoons olive oil
- 2 eggplants, chopped
- 1 brown onion, chopped
- 1 red bell pepper, chopped
- 3 garlic cloves, minced
- 1 tablespoon thyme, dried
- 2 teaspoons sage, dried
- 4 ounces canned white beans, drained
- 1 cup chicken stock
- 12 ounces zucchinis, chopped
- Salt and pepper to taste
- 2 tablespoons tomato paste

Directions

1. In a bowl, mix flour with salt, pepper, pork neck, and toss.
2. Heat a pan with 2 teaspoons oil over a medium-high heat, add pork and cook for 3 minutes on each side.
3. Transfer pork to a slow cooker and leave aside. Heat the remaining oil in the same pan over medium heat, add eggplant, onion, bell pepper, thyme, sage, and garlic, stir and cook for 5 minutes.
4. Add reserved flour, stir, and cook for 1 more minute. Add to pork, then add beans, stock, tomato paste, and zucchinis.
5. Cover and cook on High for 4 hours. Uncover, transfer to plates, and serve.

Nutritions: Calories: 310g, Fat: 31g, Fiber: 15g, Carbs: 21g, Protein: 23g

82. Gluten-Free Portobello Pesto Egg Omelet

Preparation:
10 Minutes

Cooking:
25 Minutes

Servings:
1

Ingredients

- Olive oil (1 tsp.)
- Portobello mushroom cap (1)
- Red onion (.25 cup)
- Egg whites (4)
- Water (1 tsp.)
- Black pepper & salt (to taste)
- Prepared pesto (1 tsp.)
- Shredded low-fat mozzarella cheese (.25 cup)

Directions

1. Pour and warm the oil in a skillet using the medium temperature setting.
2. Chop and add the onions and mushrooms to sauté for about three to five minutes or until they're softened.
3. Crack the eggs into a bowl and whisk in the salt, pepper, and water. Dump the eggs on top of the onions and mushrooms.
4. Continue cooking for about five minutes, stirring occasionally. Sprinkle it using the cheese and top it off with some pesto.
5. Fold the omelet in half and continue cooking for about two to three more minutes before servings.

Nutritions: *Calories: 259, Protein: 28g, Fat: 12g*

83. Feta Baked Eggs

Preparation:
5 Minutes

Cooking:
15 Minutes

Servings:
2

Directions

1. Toss butter in the skillet.
2. Add olive oil and bring it to boil.
3. After this, crack the eggs in the skillet.
4. Sprinkle them with chili flakes and onion powder.
5. Then preheat the oven to 360°F
6. Transfer the skillet with eggs to the oven and cook for 10 minutes. Then crumble feta cheese and sprinkle it over the eggs.
7. Bake the eggs for 5 minutes more
8. Top with chopped dill and serve.

Ingredients

- 1 tsp. butter
- ½ tsp. olive oil
- 2 eggs
- ¼ tsp. onion powder
- ¼ tsp. chili flakes
- 2 oz. or 57 g Feta cheese
- 1 tsp. freshly chopped dill

Nutritions: Calories: 167, Protein: 9.7g, Fat: 13.5g, Carbs: 2g

84. Easy Roasted Pork Shoulder

Preparation: 30 Minutes

Cooking: 4 Hours

Servings: 6

Ingredients

- 3 tablespoons garlic, minced
- 3 tablespoons olive oil
- 4 pounds pork shoulder
- Salt and black pepper to taste

Directions

1. In a bowl, mix olive oil with salt, pepper, and oil and whisk well.
2. Brush pork shoulder with this mix, arrange in a baking dish, and place in the oven at 425 degrees for 20 minutes.
3. Reduce heat to 325 degrees F and bake for 4 hours.
4. Take pork shoulder out of the oven, slice, and arrange on a platter. Serve with your favorite Mediterranean side salad.

Nutritions: *Calories: 224, Fat: 31g, Fiber: 15g, Carbs: 21g, Protein: 23g*

85. Herb Roasted Pork

Preparation:
20 Minutes

Cooking:
2 Hours

Servings:
10

Ingredients

- 5 and ½ pounds pork loin roast, trimmed, chine bone removed
- Salt and black pepper to taste
- 3 garlic cloves, minced
- 2 tablespoons rosemary, chopped
- 1 teaspoon fennel, ground
- 1 tablespoon fennel seeds
- 2 teaspoons red pepper, crushed
- ¼ cup olive oil

Directions

1. In a food processor mix garlic with fennel seeds, fennel, rosemary, red pepper, some black pepper, and the olive oil and blend until you obtain a paste.
2. Place pork roast in a roasting pan, spread 2 tablespoons of garlic paste all over, and rub well.
3. Season with salt and pepper, place in the oven at 400 degrees F, and bake for 1 hour.
4. Reduce heat to 325F and bake for another 35 minutes. Carve roast into chops, divide between plates, and serve right away.

Nutritions: Calories: 320, Fat: 31g, Fiber: 15g, Carbs: 21g, Protein: 23 g

86. Slow Cooked Beef Brisket

Preparation:
10 Minutes

Cooking:
9 Hours

Servings:
8

Directions

1. In a slow cooker, combine the beef with the cumin, rosemary, coriander, oregano, cinnamon, salt, pepper, and stock.
2. Cover and cook on low for 9 hours. Slice and serve.

Ingredients

- 6 pounds beef brisket
- 2 tablespoons cumin, ground
- 3 tablespoons rosemary, chopped
- 2 tablespoons coriander, dried
- 1 tablespoon oregano, dried
- 2 teaspoons cinnamon powder
- 1 cup beef stock
- A pinch of salt and black pepper

Nutritions: *Calories: 400, Fat: 31g, Fiber: 15g, Carbs: 21g, Protein: 23g*

87. Mediterranean Beef Dish

Preparation:
10 Minutes

Cooking:
15 Minutes

Servings:
6

Directions

1. Heat a pan over medium-high heat, add beef, onion, salt, pepper, and zucchini, stir, and cook for 7 minutes.
2. Add water, tomatoes, and garlic, stir, and bring to a boil. Add rice, more salt, and pepper, stir, cover, take off the heat and leave aside for 7 minutes.
3. Divide between plates and serve with cheddar cheese on top.

Ingredients

- 1-pound beef, ground
- 2 cups zucchinis, chopped
- ½ cup yellow onion, chopped
- Salt and black pepper to taste
- 15 ounces canned roasted tomatoes and garlic
- 1 cup water
- ¾ cup cheddar cheese, shredded
- 1 and ½ cups white rice

Nutritions: Calories: 320, Fat: 31g, Fiber: 15g, Carbs: 21g, Protein: 23g

88. Beef Tartare

Preparation:
10 Minutes

Cooking:
20 Minutes

Servings:
1

Directions

1. In a bowl, mix meat with shallot, egg yolk, salt, pepper, mustard, cucumbers, and parsley.
2. Stir well and arrange on a platter.
3. Garnish with the chopped parsley sprig and serve.

Ingredients

- 1 shallot, chopped
- 4 ounces beef fillet, minced
- 5 small cucumbers, chopped
- 1 egg yolk
- A pinch of salt and black pepper
- 2 teaspoons mustard
- 1 tablespoon parsley, chopped
- 1 parsley sprig, roughly chopped for serving

Nutritions: *Calories: 244, Fat: 31g, Fiber: 15g, Carbs: 21g, Protein: 23g*

89. Meatballs and Sauce

Preparation:
5 Minutes

Cooking:
8 Minutes

Servings:
4

Directions

1. In a bowl, mix the beef with the breadcrumbs, egg, cumin, allspice, cilantro, salt, and pepper.
2. Stir well and shape into medium-sized meatballs. Heat a pan with oil over medium heat.
3. Add the meatballs and cook for 4 minutes on each side. In a bowl, mix the yogurt with the cucumber, lemon juice, and dill - whisk well. Serve the meatballs with the yogurt sauce.

Ingredients

- 1 egg, whisked
- 1 teaspoon cumin, ground
- 1 teaspoon allspice, ground
- ¼ cup cilantro, chopped
- A pinch of salt and black pepper
- 2 pounds beef, ground
- ⅓ cup breadcrumbs
- Vegetable oil for frying
- For the sauce:
- 1 cucumber, chopped
- 1 cup Greek yogurt
- 2 tablespoons lemon juice
- 1 tablespoon dill, chopped

Nutritions: Calories: 263, Fat: 31g, Fiber: 15g, Carbs: 21g, Protein: 23g

90. Poached Eggs

Preparation:
10 Minutes

Cooking:
10 Minutes

Servings:
2

Ingredients

- Salt (.5 tsp.)
- Champagne vinegar (1 tsp.)
- Fresh eggs (2)

Directions

1. Prepare a cooking pot with cold water. Wait for it to boil using the medium temperature setting. Stir in the salt and vinegar.
2. Break each of the eggs into a ramekin. Place it close to the water and slide it out of the dish. Simmer until set.
3. Use a slotted spoon to lift it from the pan to help prevent sticking. Continue cooking until the yolk is runny and the white is cooked or about six minutes.
4. Prepare a container with ice water. Place the eggs into the bowl of ice water (it slows and stops the cooking process.)
5. Put them in paper towels to remove the water and serve.

Nutritions: *Calories: 72, Protein: 6.3g, Fat: 5g*

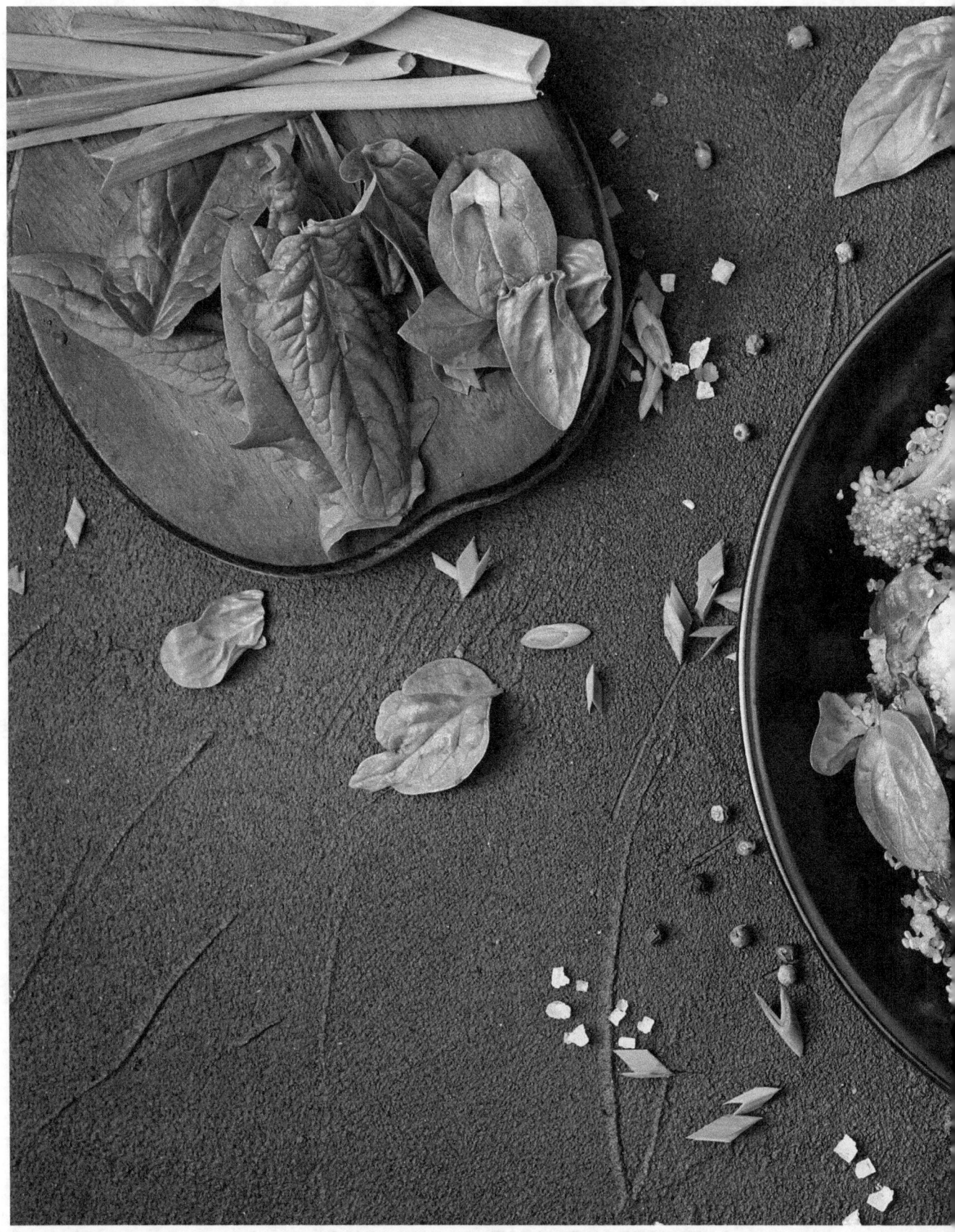

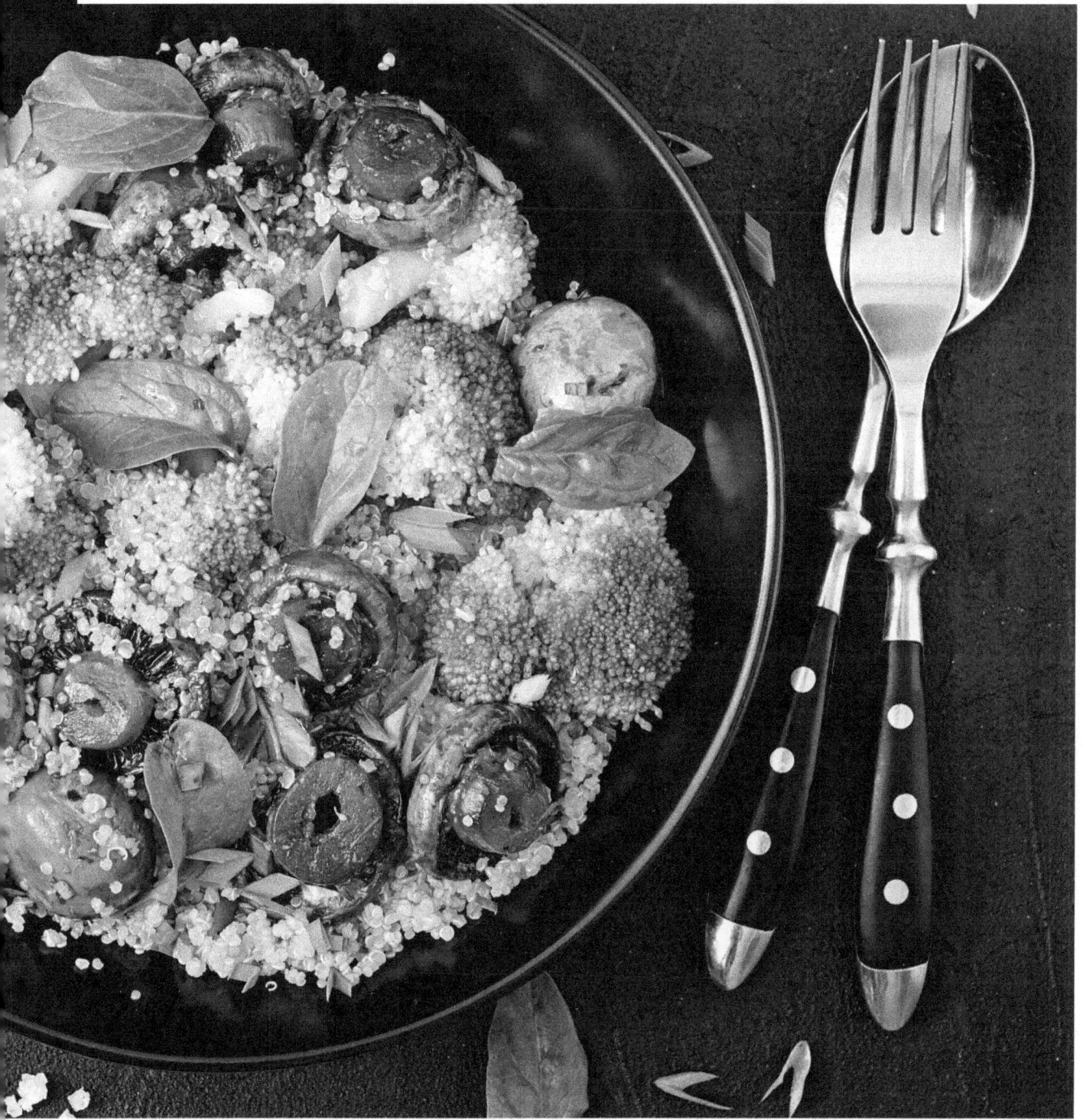

CHAPTER 14:
Vegetarian Recipes

91. Roasted Vegetables and Chickpeas

Preparation:
15 Minutes

Cooking:
30 Minutes

Servings:
2

Ingredients

- 4 cups cauliflower florets
- 2 medium carrots, sliced into quarters
- 2 tbsp olive oil, divided
- ½ tsp garlic powder, divided
- ½ tsp salt, divided
- 2 tsp zaatar spice mix, divided
- 1 can chickpeas, patted dry
- ¾ cup plain Greek yogurt
- 1 tsp harissa spice paste

Directions

1. Warm-up the oven to 400 F.
2. Arrange a sheet pan with parchment paper.
3. Put the cauliflower and carrots in a bowl, add 1 tablespoon olive oil, ¼ teaspoon of garlic powder, ¼ teaspoon of salt, and 1 teaspoon zaatar. Toss well to combine.
4. Put the vegetables onto half of the sheet pan in a single layer.
5. Put the chickpeas in the same bowl and season with the remaining 1 tablespoon of oil, ¼ teaspoon of garlic powder, and ¼ teaspoon of salt, and the remaining za'atar. Toss well to combine.
6. Put the chickpeas onto the other half of the sheet pan.
7. Roast within 30 minutes. Flip it halfway through the cooking time, and stir the chickpeas, so they cook evenly.
8. In the meantime, mix the yogurt and harissa in a bowl. Then serve.

Nutritions: Calories: 468, Fat: 23.0g, Protein: 18.1g, Carbs: 54.1g, Fiber: 13.8g, Sodium: 631mg

92. Veggie Rice Bowls with Pesto Sauce

Preparation:
15 Minutes

Cooking:
1 Minutes

Servings:
2

Ingredients

- 2 cups of water
- 1 cup arborio rice, rinsed
- Salt and ground black pepper, to taste
- 2 eggs
- 1 cup broccoli florets
- ½ pound (227g) Brussels sprouts
- 1 carrot, peeled and chopped
- 1 small beet, peeled and cubed
- ¼ cup pesto sauce
- Lemon wedges, for serving

Directions

1. Combine the water, rice, salt, and pepper in the Instant Pot. Insert a trivet over rice and place a steamer basket on top.
2. Add the eggs, broccoli, Brussels sprouts, carrots, beet cubes, salt, and pepper to the steamer basket.
3. Lock the lid. Select the Manual mode and set the cooking time for 1 minute at High Pressure.
4. When the timer beeps, perform a natural pressure release for 10 minutes, then release any remaining pressure. Carefully open the lid.
5. Remove the steamer basket and trivet from the pot and transfer the eggs to a bowl of ice water. Peel and halve the eggs. Use a fork to fluff the rice.
6. Divide the rice, broccoli, Brussels sprouts, carrot, beet cubes, and eggs into two bowls. Top with a dollop of pesto sauce and serve with the lemon wedges.

Nutritions: *Calories: 590, Fat: 34.1g, Protein: 21.9g, Carbs: 50.0g, Fiber: 19.6g, Sodium: 670mg*

93. Sautéed Spinach and Leeks

Preparation:
5 Minutes

Cooking:
8 Minutes

Servings:
2

Directions

1. Oil the bottom of the pot with the olive oil.
2. Add the garlic, leek, and onions and stir-fry for about 5 minutes on Sauté mode.
3. Stir in the spinach. Sprinkle with the salt and sauté for an additional 3 minutes, stirring constantly.
4. Transfer to a plate and scatter with the goat cheese before serving.

Ingredients

- 3 tablespoons olive oil
- 2 garlic cloves, crushed
- 2 leeks, chopped
- 2 red onions, chopped
- 9 ounces (255g) fresh spinach
- 1 teaspoon kosher salt
- ½ cup crumbled goat cheese

Nutritions: Calories: 447, Fat: 31.2g, Protein: 14.6g, Carbs: 28.7g, Fiber: 6.3g, Sodium: 937mg

94. Vegan Sesame Tofu and Eggplants

Preparation:
10 Minutes

Cooking:
20 Minutes

Servings:
4

Ingredients

- 5 tablespoons olive oil
- 1-pound firm tofu, sliced
- 3 tablespoons rice vinegar
- 2 teaspoons Swerve sweetener
- 2 whole eggplants, sliced
- ¼ cup soy sauce
- Salt and pepper to taste
- 4 tablespoons toasted sesame oil
- ¼ cup sesame seeds
- 1 cup fresh cilantro, chopped

Directions

1. Heat the oil in a pan for 2 minutes.
2. Pan-fry the tofu for 3 minutes on each side.
3. Stir in the rice vinegar, sweetener, eggplants, and soy sauce. Season with salt and pepper to taste.
4. Cover and cook for 5 minutes on medium fire. Stir and continue cooking for another 5 minutes.
5. Toss in the sesame oil, sesame seeds, and cilantro.
6. Serve and enjoy.

Nutritions: *Calories: 616, Carbs: 27.4g, Protein: 23.9g, Fat: 49.2g*

95. Vegetarian Coconut Curry

Preparation:
10 Minutes

Cooking:
30 Minutes

Servings:
4

Directions

1. Heat oil in a pot.
2. Sauté the onion and garlic until fragrant, around 3 minutes.
3. Stir in the rest of the ingredients, except for spinach leaves.
4. Season with salt and pepper to taste.
5. Cover and cook on medium fire for 5 minutes.
6. Stir and add spinach leaves. Cover and cook for another 2 minutes.
7. Turn off the fire and let it sit for two more minutes before serving.

Ingredients

- 4 tablespoons coconut oil
- 1 medium onion, chopped
- 1 teaspoon minced garlic
- 1 teaspoon minced ginger
- 1 cup broccoli florets
- 2 cups fresh spinach leaves
- 2 teaspoons fish sauce
- 1 tablespoon garam masala
- ½ cup coconut milk
- Salt and pepper to taste

Nutritions: Calories: 210, Carbs: 6.5g, Protein: 2.1g, Fat: 20.9g

96. Zoodles with Beet Pesto

Preparation: 10 Minutes

Cooking: 50 Minutes

Servings: 2

Ingredients

- 1 medium red beet, chopped
- ½ cup walnut pieces
- ½ cup crumbled goat cheese
- 3 garlic cloves
- 2 tbsp freshly squeezed lemon juice
- 2 tbsp + 2 tsp extra-virgin olive oil, divided
- ¼ tsp salt
- 4 small zucchinis, spiralized

Directions

1. Warm-up the oven to 375 F.
2. Cover the chopped beet with aluminum foil and seal well.
3. Roast in the oven within 30 to 40 minutes until tender.
4. In the meantime, warm a skillet over medium-high heat, then put in the walnuts and toast for 5 to 7 minutes, or until fragrant and lightly browned.
5. Put the cooked beets in a food processor. Add the toasted walnuts, goat cheese, garlic, lemon juice, 2 tablespoons of olive oil, and salt. Pulse until smoothly blended. Set aside.
6. Heat the remaining 2 teaspoons of olive oil in a large skillet over medium heat. Put the zucchini and toss to coat in the oil. Cook within 2 to 3 minutes, stirring gently, or until the zucchini is softened.
7. Transfer the toss with th

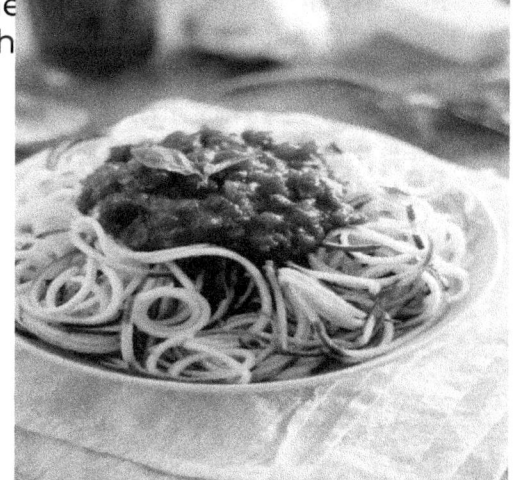

Nutritions: *Calories: 423, Fat: 38.8g, Protein: 8.0g, Carbs: 17.1g, Fiber: 6.0g, Sodium: 338mg*

97. Sweet Potato Chickpea Buddha Bowl

Preparation:
10 Minutes

Cooking:
15 Minutes

Servings:
2

Ingredients

Sauce:
- 1 tablespoon tahini
- 2 tablespoons plain Greek yogurt
- 2 tablespoons hemp seeds
- 1 garlic clove, minced
- Pinch salt
- Freshly ground black pepper, to taste

Bowl:
- 1 small sweet potato, diced
- 1 tsp extra-virgin olive oil
- 1 cup low-sodium chickpeas, drained and rinsed
- 2 cups baby kale

Directions

1. Make the Sauce:
2. Whisk the tahini and yogurt in a small bowl.
3. Stir in the hemp seeds and minced garlic, then season with salt pepper. Add 2 to 3 tablespoons water to create a creamy yet pourable consistency and set aside.
4. Make the Bowl:
5. Preheat the oven to 425°F (220°C).
6. Put the sweet potato on the baking sheet and drizzle with the olive oil. Toss well
7. Roast in the oven for 10 to 15 minutes, stirring once during cooking, or until fork-tender and browned.
8. In both of the bowls, place ½ cup of chickpeas, 1 cup of baby kale, and half of the cooked sweet potato. Serve drizzled with half of the prepared sauce.

Nutritions: Calories: 323, Fat: 14.1g, Protein: 17.0g, Carbs: 36.0 g, Fiber: 7.9g, Sodium: 304mg

98. Easy Zucchini Patties

Preparation:
15 Minutes

Cooking:
5 Minutes

Servings:
2

Ingredients

- 2 medium zucchinis, shredded
- 1 teaspoon salt, divided
- 2 eggs
- 2 tablespoons chickpea flour
- 1 tablespoon chopped fresh mint
- 1 scallion, chopped
- 2 tablespoons extra-virgin olive oil

Directions

1. Put the shredded zucchini in a fine-mesh strainer and season with ½ teaspoon of salt. Set aside.
2. Beat the eggs, chickpea flour, mint, scallion, and remaining ½ teaspoon of salt in a medium bowl.
3. Squeeze the zucchini to drain as much liquid as possible. Add the zucchini to the egg mixture and stir until well incorporated.
4. Warm-up the olive oil in a skillet over medium-high heat.
5. Drop the zucchini mixture by spoonsful into the skillet. Gently flatten the zucchini with the back of a spatula.
6. Cook for 2 to 3 minutes or until golden brown. Flip and cook for an additional 2 minutes. Serve.

Nutritions: *Calories: 264, Fat: 20.0g, Protein: 9.8g, Carbs: 16.1g, Fiber: 4.0g, Sodium: 1780mg*

99. Zucchini Crisp

Preparation:
10 Minutes

Cooking:
20 Minutes

Servings:
2

Ingredients

- 4 zucchinis, sliced into ½-inch rounds
- ½ cup unsweetened almond milk
- 1 teaspoon fresh lemon juice
- 1 teaspoon arrowroot powder
- ½ teaspoon salt, divided
- ½ cup whole wheat breadcrumbs
- ¼ cup nutritional yeast
- ¼ cup hemp seeds
- ½ teaspoon garlic powder
- ¼ teaspoon crushed red pepper
- ¼ teaspoon black pepper

Directions

1. Warm-up the oven to 375 F. Line two baking sheets with parchment paper and set aside.
2. Put the zucchini in a medium bowl with the almond milk, lemon juice, arrowroot powder, and ¼ teaspoon salt. Stir to mix well.
3. In a large bowl, thoroughly combine the breadcrumbs, nutritional yeast, hemp seeds, garlic powder, crushed red pepper, and black pepper.
4. Add the zucchini in batches and shake until the slices are evenly coated. Put the zucchini on the baking sheets in a single layer.
5. Bake in the preheated oven for about 20 minutes, or until the zucchini slices are golden brown.
6. Season with the remaining ¼ teaspoon of salt before serving.

Nutritions: Calories: 255, Fat: 11.3g, Protein: 8.6g, Carbs: 31.9g, Fiber: 3.8g, Sodium: 826mg

CHAPTER 15:
Sandwiches and Wraps

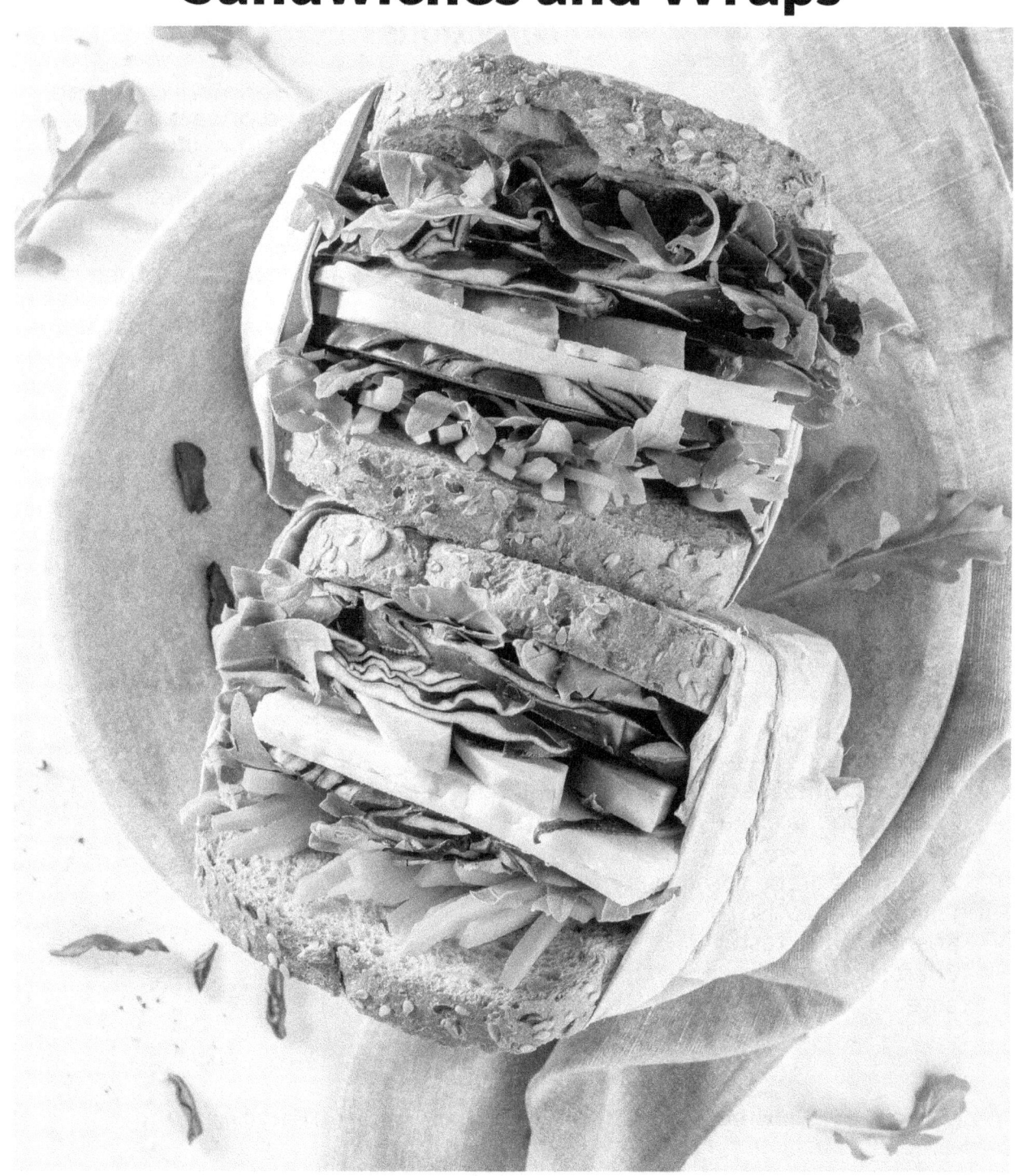

100. Mediterranean Egg White Breakfast Sandwich

Preparation:
10 Minutes

Cooking:
25 Minutes

Servings:
2

Ingredients

- 2 teaspoons butter
- Salt to taste
- Pepper to taste
- 2 whole-grain seeded ciabatta rolls, split, toasted
- 2 slices Swiss cheese or Muenster cheese
- ½ cup egg whites, beaten
- 2 teaspoon minced fresh herbs of your choice
- 2 tablespoons pesto

For roasted tomatoes:
- 2 tablespoons extra-virgin olive oil
- 20 ounces grape tomatoes, halved lengthwise
- Kosher salt to taste
- Coarsely ground pepper to taste

Directions

1. Heat a nonstick pan over medium flame.
2. Toss half the butter and once it starts melting, add half the egg whites.
3. Sprinkle salt, pepper, and 1 teaspoon of herbs, and cook until the omelet is set. Flip sides and cook the other side for about 30 seconds. Place onto a plate.
4. Repeat steps 2-3 and make the other omelet.
5. Meanwhile, make the roasted tomatoes as follows: Add tomatoes into a baking dish. Pour oil over it and toss well. Sprinkle with salt and pepper. Spread it evenly in the dish.
6. Roast in a preheated oven at 400° F for about 20 minutes or until charred slightly.
7. Toast the rolls just before serving.
8. Spread pesto on the cut part of the rolls.
9. Place bottom halves of the rolls on individual serving plates. Place an omelet on each, folding it to fit it in.
10. Place a slice of cheese on each. Cover with the top half of the rolls and serve.

Nutritions: Calories 468, Protein 14.0g, Carbs: 4.0g, Fat: 20.0g

101. Mediterranean Lettuce Wraps

Preparation:
10 Minutes

Cooking:
10 Minutes

Servings:
4

Ingredients

- ¼ cup of tahini
- ¼ cup of olive oil, extra-virgin
- 1 teaspoon of lemon zest
- ¼ cup of lemon juice
- 1½ tsp. of pure maple syrup
- ¾ tsp. of kosher salt
- ½ tsp. of paprika
- 2 cans (15 ounces) of rinsed chickpeas, no-salt-added
- ½ cup of sliced and roasted red pepper - drained and jarred
- ½ cup of thinly sliced shallots
- 12 leaves of Bibb lettuce, large
- ¼ cup of almonds, roasted and chopped
- 2 tsp. of fresh parsley, chopped

Directions

1. Whisk lemon zest, tahini, oil, maple syrup, lemon juice, paprika, and all in a bowl.
2. After this, add peppers, chickpeas, and shallots.
3. Toss for coating.
4. After this, divide this mixture among the lettuce leaves (say about one-third cup for every portion).
5. Top with parsley and almonds.
6. Before serving, wrap lettuce leaves around this filling for proper garnishing.

Nutritions: *Carbohydrate: 44g, Protein: 16g, Fat: 28g, Calories: 498*

102. Shrimp, Avocado, and Feta Wrap

Preparation:
5 Minutes

Cooking:
5 Minutes

Servings:
2

Ingredients

- Chopped cooked shrimp (3 ounces)
- Lime juice (1 tablespoon)
- Crumbled feta cheese (2 tablespoons)
- Diced avocado (¼ cup)
- Whole-wheat tortilla (1 piece)
- Diced tomato (¼ cup)
- Sliced scallion (1 Piece)

Directions

1. Spray vegetable oil on a skillet and then heat it. Add the shrimp to get a nice pink color to them.
2. Add the feta cheese on one side of the wrap and also be generous with the cheese.
3. Top the cheese with the various other ingredients. Add the shrimp on the top so they will be in the middle of the wrap when you roll it.
4. Add lime juice to give it the tangy zing to the wrap.
5. Then roll the wrap tightly, but make sure that the ingredients don't fall off.
6. Then cut the wrap in two halves and serve it.

Nutritions: Carbohydrate: 34g, Protein: 29g, Fat: 14g, Calories: 371

103. Flatbread Sandwiches

Preparation:
5 Minutes

Cooking:
10 Minutes

Servings:
6

Directions

1. Cook the pilaf as directed on the package instructions and cool.
2. Chop and combine the tomato, cucumber, cheese, oil, pepper, and lemon juice. Fold in the pilaf.
3. Prepare the wraps with the hummus on one side. Spoon in the pilaf and fold.
4. Slice into a sandwich and serve.

Ingredients

- Olive oil (1 tbsp.)
- 7-grain pilaf (8.5 oz. pkg.)
- English seedless cucumber (1 cup)
- Seeded tomato (1 cup)
- Crumbled feta cheese (.25 cup)
- Fresh lemon juice (2 tbsp.)
- Freshly cracked black pepper (.25 tsp.)
- Plain hummus (7 oz. container)
- Whole grain white flatbread wraps (threeat 2.8 oz. each)

Nutritions: Calories: 310, Protein: 10g, Fat: 9g

104. Bean Lettuce Wraps

Preparation:
5 Minutes

Cooking:
20 Minutes

Servings:
4

Ingredients

- 8 romaine lettuce leaves
- ½ cup garlic hummus or any prepared hummus
- ¾ cup chopped tomatoes
- 15 ounce can great northern beans, drained and rinsed
- ½ cup diced onion
- 1 tablespoon extra-virgin olive oil
- ¼ cup chopped parsley
- ¼ teaspoon black pepper

Directions

1. Set a skillet on top of the stove range over medium heat.
2. In the skillet, warm the oil for a couple of minutes.
3. Add the onion to the oil. Stir frequently as the onion cooks for a few minutes.
4. Combine the pepper and tomatoes and cook for another couple of minutes. Remember to stir occasionally.
5. Add the beans and continue to stir and cook for 2 to 3 minutes.
6. Turn the burner off, remove the skillet from heat, and add the parsley.
7. Set the lettuce leaves on a flat surface and spread 1 tablespoon of hummus on each leaf.
8. Divide the bean mixture onto the 8 leaves.
9. Spread the bean mixture down the center of the leaves.
10. Fold the leaves by starting lengthwise on one side.
11. Fold over the other side so the leaf is completely wrapped.
12. Serve and enjoy.

Nutritions: Calories: 211, Fats: 8g, Carbohydrates: 28g, Protein: 10g

105. Italian Tuna Sandwiches

Preparation: 10 Minutes

Cooking: 0 Minutes

Servings: 4

Ingredients

- 3 tablespoons freshly squeezed lemon juice
- 2 tablespoons extra-virgin olive oil
- 1 garlic clove, minced
- ½ teaspoon freshly ground black pepper
- 2 (5-ounce) cans tuna, drained
- 1 (2.25-ounce) can sliced olives
- ½ cup chopped fresh fennel, including fronds
- 8 slices whole-grain crusty bread

Directions

1. In a medium bowl, whisk to combine the lemon juice, oil, garlic, and pepper. Add the tuna, olives, and fennel. Using a fork, separate the tuna into chunks and stir to combine all the ingredients.
2. Divide the tuna salad equally among 4 slices of bread. Top each with the remaining bread slices. Let the sandwiches sit for at least 5 minutes so the zesty filling can soak into the bread before serving.

Nutritions: *Calories: 347, Fat: 17g, Fiber: 5g, Protein: 25g*

106. Dill Salmon Salad Wraps

Preparation:
10 Minutes

Cooking:
10 Minutes

Servings:
6

Directions

1. In a large bowl, mix together the salmon, carrots, celery, dill, red onion, capers, oil, vinegar, pepper, and salt. Divide the salmon salad among the flatbreads. Fold up the bottom of the flatbread, then roll up the wrap and serve.

Ingredients

- 1-pound salmon filet, cooked and flaked
- ½ cup diced carrots
- ½ cup diced celery
- 3 tablespoons chopped fresh dill
- 3 tablespoons diced red onion
- 2 tablespoons capers
- 1½ tablespoons extra-virgin olive oil
- 1 tablespoon aged balsamic vinegar
- ½ teaspoon freshly ground black pepper
- ¼ teaspoon kosher or sea salt
- 4 whole-wheat flatbread wraps or soft whole-wheat tortillas

Nutritions: Calories: 336, Fat: 16g, Fiber: 5g, Protein: 32g

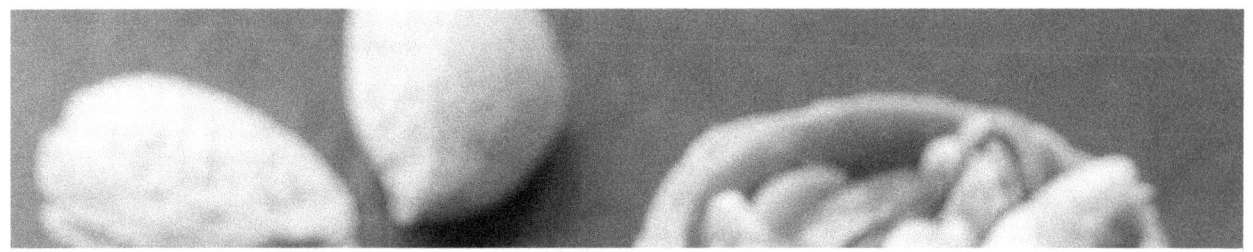

CHAPTER 16:
Desserts and Fruits

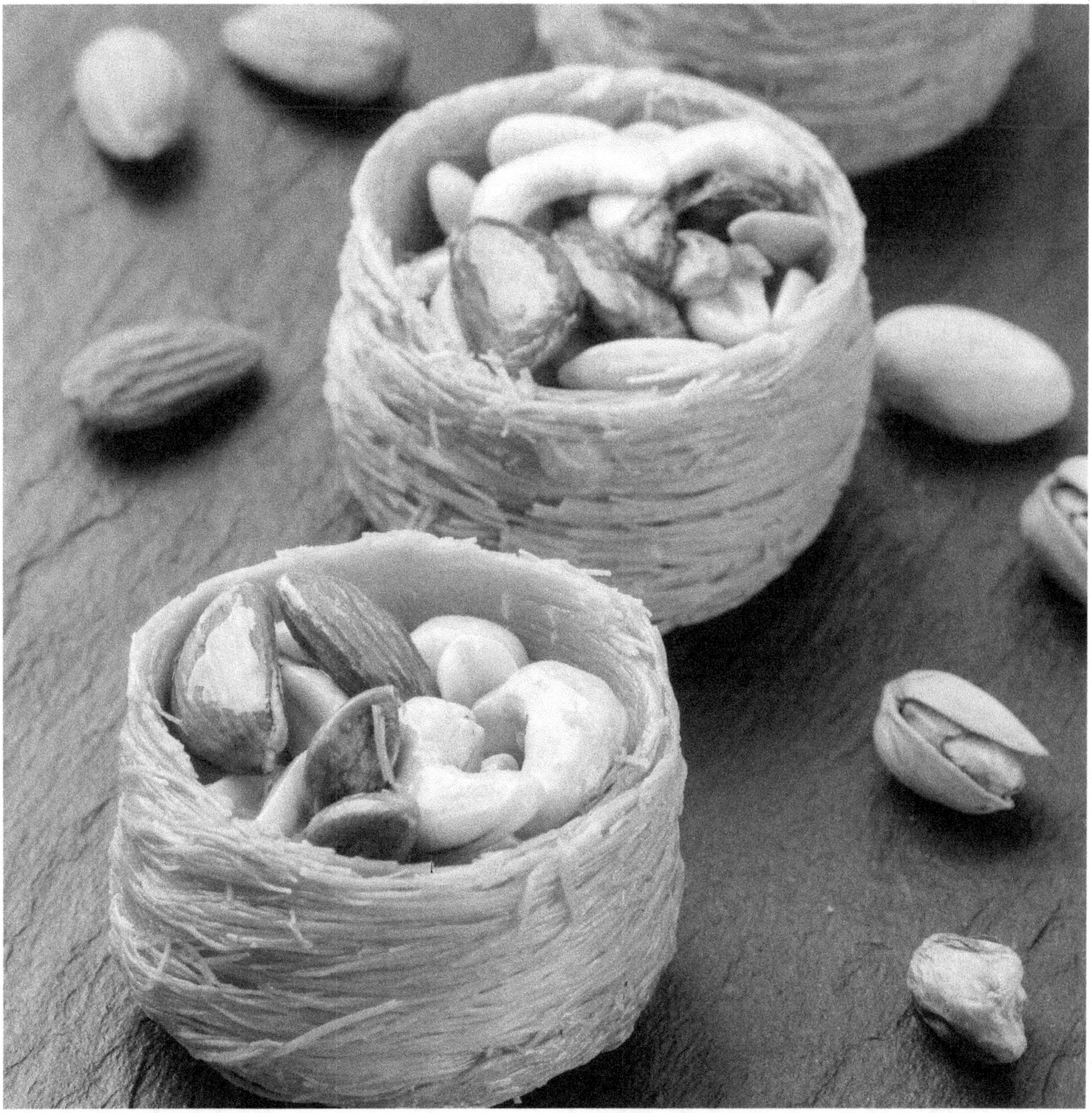

107. Mascarpone and Fig Crostini

Preparation:
10 Minutes

Cooking:
10 Minutes

Servings:
6-8

Ingredients

- 1 long French baguette
- 4 tablespoons (½ stick) salted butter, melted
- 1 (8-ounce) tub mascarpone cheese
- 1 (12-ounce) jar fig jam or preserves

Directions

1. Preheat the oven to 350°F.
2. Slice the bread into ¼-inch-thick slices.
3. Lay out the sliced bread on a single baking sheet and brush each slice with the melted butter.
4. Put the single baking sheet in the oven and toast the bread for 5 to 7 minutes until golden brown.
5. Let the bread cool slightly. Spread it with a teaspoon or so of the mascarpone cheese on each piece of the bread.
6. Top with a teaspoon or so of the jam. Serve immediately.

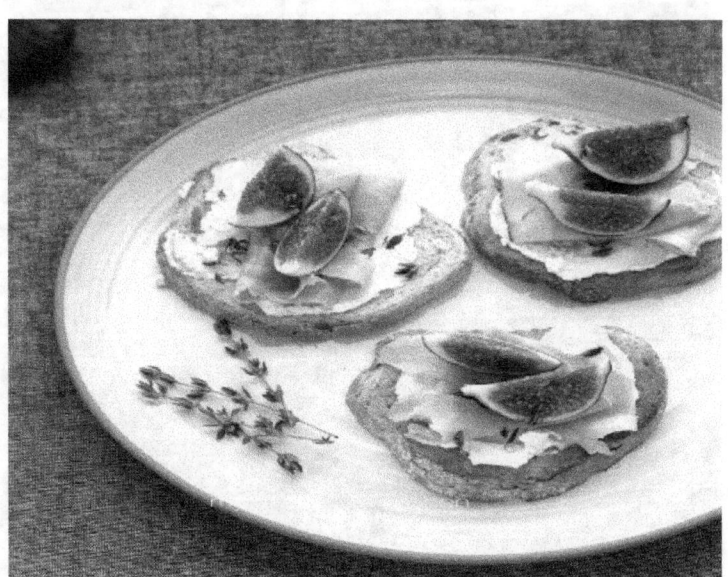

Nutritions: Calories: 445, Fat: 24g, Carbs: 48g, Protein: 3g

108. Crunchy Sesame Cookies

Preparation:
10 Minutes

Cooking:
15 Minutes

Servings:
14-16

Ingredients

- 1 cup sesame seeds, hulled
- 1 cup sugar
- 8 tablespoons (1 stick) salted butter, softened
- 2 large eggs
- 1¼ cups flour

Directions

1. Preheat the oven to 350°F. Toast the sesame seeds on a baking sheet for 3 minutes. Set aside and leave to cool.
2. Using a mixer, cream together the sugar and butter.
3. Put the eggs in one at a time until well-blended.
4. Add the flour and toasted sesame seeds and mix until well-blended.
5. Drop spoonfuls of cookie dough onto a baking sheet and form them into round balls, about 1-inch in diameter, similar to a walnut.
6. Put in the oven and bake for 5 to 7 minutes or until golden brown.
7. Let the cookies cool and enjoy.

Nutritions: *Calories: 218, Fat: 12g, Carbs: 25g, Protein: 4g*

109. Almond Cookies

Preparation:
5 Minutes

Cooking:
10 Minutes

Servings:
4-6

Ingredients

- ½ cup sugar
- 8 tablespoons (1 stick) room temperature salted butter
- 1 large egg
- 1½ cups all-purpose flour
- 1 cup ground almonds or almond flour

Directions

1. Preheat the oven to 375°F.
2. Using a mixer, cream together the sugar and butter.
3. Add the egg and mix until combined.
4. Alternately add the flour and ground almonds, ½ cup at a time, while the mixer is on slow.
5. Once everything is combined, line a baking sheet with parchment paper. Drop a tablespoon of dough on the baking sheet, keeping the cookies at least 2 inches apart.
6. Put the single baking sheet in the oven and bake just until the cookies start to turn brown around the edges for about 5 to 7 minutes.

Nutritions: Calories: 604, Fat: 36g, Carbs: 63g, Protein: 11g

110. Baklava and Honey

Preparation:
40 Minutes

Cooking:
1 Hour

Servings:
6-8

Ingredients

- 2 cups chopped walnuts or pecans
- 1 teaspoon cinnamon
- 1 cup of melted unsalted butter
- 1 (16-ounce) package phyllo dough, thawed
- 1 (12-ounce) jar honey

Directions

1. Preheat the oven to 350°F.
2. In a bowl, combine the chopped nuts and cinnamon.
3. Using a brush, butter the sides and bottom of a 9-by-13-inch baking dish.
4. Take off the phyllo dough from the package and cut it to the size of the baking dish using a sharp knife.
5. Put one sheet of phyllo dough on the bottom of the dish, brush with butter, and repeat until you have 8 layers.
6. Sprinkle ⅓ cup of the nut mixture over the phyllo layers. Top with a sheet of phyllo dough, butter that sheet, and repeat until you have 4 sheets of buttered phyllo dough.
7. Sprinkle ⅓ cup of the nut mixture for another layer of nuts. Repeat the layering of nuts and 4 sheets of buttered phyllo until all the nut mixture is gone. The last layer should be 8 buttered sheets of phyllo.
8. Before you bake, cut the baklava into desired shapes; traditionally this is diamonds, triangles, or squares.
9. Bake the baklava for about 1 hour just until the top layer is golden brown.
10. While the baklava is baking, heat the honey in a pan just until it is warm and easy to pour.
11. Once the baklava is done baking, directly pour the honey evenly over the baklava and let it absorb it, about 20 minutes. Serve warm or at room temperature.

Nutritions: *Calories: 1235, Fat: 89g, Carbs: 109g, Protein: 18g*

111. Date and Nut Balls

Preparation:
10 Minutes

Cooking:
10 Minutes

Servings:
6-8

Ingredients

- 1 cup walnuts or pistachios
- 1 cup unsweetened shredded coconut
- 14 Medjool dates, pits removed
- 8 tablespoons (1 stick) butter, melted

Directions

1. Preheat the oven to 350°F.
2. Put the nuts on a baking sheet. Toast the nuts for 5 minutes.
3. Put the shredded coconut on a clean baking sheet; toast just until it turns golden brown, about 3 to 5 minutes (coconut burns fast so keep an eye on it). Once done, remove it from the oven and put it in a shallow bowl.
4. Inside a food processor with a chopping blade, put the nuts until they have a medium chop. Put the chopped nuts into a medium bowl.
5. Add the dates and melted butter to the food processor and blend until the dates become a thick paste. Pour the chopped nuts into the food processor with the dates and pulse just until the mixture is combined, about 5 to 7 pulses.
6. Remove the mixture from the food processor and scrape it into a large bowl.
7. To make the balls, spoon 1 to 2 tablespoons of the date mixture into the palm of your hand and roll around between your hands until you form a ball. Put the ball on a clean, lined baking sheet. Repeat this until all of the mixture is formed into balls.
8. Roll each ball in the toasted coconut until the outside of the ball is coated, put the ball back on the baking sheet, and repeat.
9. Put all the balls into the fridge for 20 minutes before serving so that they firm up. You can also store any leftovers inside the fridge in an airtight container.

Nutritions: Calories: 489, Fat: 35g, Carbs: 48g, Protein: 5g

112. Mango Snow

Preparation:
5 Minutes

Cooking:
2 Hours

Servings:
8

Ingredients

- 4 cups frozen mango in pieces
- 1 can of condensed milk (14 ounces/396 g)
- 1 can of evaporated milk (12 ounces /340 g)
- Mint leaves (decoration)
- Cookies (decoration)

Directions

1. Blend the mango, the condensed milk, and the evaporated milk at high speed for 5 minutes.
2. Transfer the mixture to the mixing bowl. Cover and leave to cool for at least 2 hours in the freezer.
3. Garnish with mint leaves and cookies.

Nutritions: *Calories: 411, Carbohydrates: 84g, Protein: 1g, Fat: 8g*

113. Minty Coconut Cream

Preparation:
4 Minutes

Cooking:
0 Minutes

Servings:
2

Directions

1. In a blender, combine the coconut with the banana and the rest of the ingredients, pulse well, divide into cups and serve cold.

Ingredients

- 1 banana, peeled
- 2 cups coconut flesh, shredded
- 3 tablespoons mint, chopped
- 1 and ½ cups coconut water
- 2 tablespoons stevia
- ½ avocado, pitted and peeled

Nutritions: Calories 193, Fat: 5.4g, Fiber: 3.4g, Carbs: 7.6g, Protein: 3g

114. Watermelon Cream

Preparation:
15 Minutes

Cooking:
0 Minutes

Servings:
2

Directions

1. In a blender, combine the watermelon with the cream and the rest of the ingredients, pulse well, divide into cups and keep in the fridge for 15 minutes before serving.

Ingredients

- 1-pound watermelon, peeled and chopped
- 1 teaspoon vanilla extract
- 1 cup heavy cream
- 1 teaspoon lime juice
- 2 tablespoons stevia

Nutritions: *Calories 122, Fat: 5.7g, Fiber: 3.2g, Carbs: 5.3g, Protein: 0.4g*

115. Grapes Stew

Preparation:
10 Minutes

Cooking:
10 Minutes

Servings:
4

Directions

1. Heat up a pan with the water over medium heat, add the oil, stevia, and the rest of the ingredients, toss, simmer for 10 minutes, divide into cups, and serve.

Ingredients

- 2/3 cup stevia
- 1 tablespoon olive oil
- ⅓ cup coconut water
- 1 teaspoon vanilla extract
- 1 teaspoon lemon zest, grated
- 2 cup red grapes, halved

Nutritions: Calories: 122, Fat: 3.7g, Fiber: 1.2g, Carbs: 2.3g, Protein: 0.4g

116. Cocoa Sweet Cherry Cream

Preparation: 2 Hours

Cooking: 0 Minutes

Servings: 4

Directions

1. In a blender, mix the cherries with the water and the rest of the ingredients, pulse well, divide into cups, and keep in the fridge for 2 hours before serving.

Ingredients

- ½ cup cocoa powder
- ¾ cup red cherry jam
- ¼ cup stevia
- 2 cups water
- 1-pound cherries, pitted and halved

Nutritions: *Calories: 162, Fat: 3.4g, Fiber: 2.4g, Carbs: 5g, Protein: 1g*

117. Creamy Rice Pudding

Preparation:
5 Minutes

Cooking:
45 Minutes

Servings:
6

Ingredients

- 1¼ cups long-grain rice
- 5 cups whole milk
- 1 cup sugar
- 1 tablespoon of rose water/ orange blossom water
- 1 teaspoon cinnamon

Directions

1. Rinse the rice under cold water for 30 seconds.
2. Add the rice, milk, and sugar to a large pot. Bring to a gentle boil while continually stirring.
3. Lessen the heat to low and then let simmer for 40 to 45 minutes, stirring every 3 to 4 minutes so that the rice does not stick to the bottom of the pot.
4. Add the rose water at the end and simmer for 5 minutes.
5. Divide the pudding into 6 bowls. Sprinkle the top with cinnamon. Let it cool for over an hour before serving. Store in the fridge.

Nutritions: Calories: 394, Fat: 7g, Carbs: 75g, Protein: 9g

118. Ricotta-Lemon Cheesecake

Preparation:
5 Minutes

Cooking:
1 Hour

Servings:
8-10

Ingredients

- 2 (8-ounce) packages full-fat cream cheese
- 1 (16-ounce) container full-fat ricotta cheese
- 1½ cups granulated sugar
- 1 tablespoon lemon zest
- 5 large eggs
- Nonstick cooking spray

Directions

1. Preheat the oven to 350°F.
2. Blend together the cream cheese and ricotta cheese.
3. Blend in the sugar and lemon zest.
4. Blend in the eggs; drop in 1 egg at a time, blend for 10 seconds, and repeat.
5. Put a 9-inch springform pan with parchment paper and nonstick spray. Wrap the bottom of the pan with foil. Pour the cheesecake batter into the pan.
6. To make a water bath, get a baking or roasting pan larger than the cheesecake pan. Fill the roasting pan about ⅓ of the way up with warm water. Put the cheesecake pan into the water bath. Put the whole thing in the oven and let the cheesecake bake for 1 hour.
7. After baking is complete, remove the cheesecake pan from the water bath and remove the foil. Let the cheesecake cool for 1 hour on the countertop. Then put it in the fridge to cool for at least 3 hours before serving.

Nutritions: *Calories: 489, Fat: 31g, Carbs: 42g, Protein: 15g*

119. Crockpot Keto Chocolate Cake

Preparation:
20 Minutes

Cooking:
3 Hours

Servings:
12

Directions

1. Grease the ceramic insert of the Crock-Pot.
2. In a bowl, mix the sweetener, almond flour, protein powder, cocoa powder, salt, and baking powder.
3. Add the butter, eggs, cream, and vanilla extract.
4. Pour the batter into the Crock-Pot and cook on low for 3 hours.
5. Allow to cool before slicing.

Ingredients

- ¾ c. stevia sweetener
- 1 ½ c. almond flour
- ¼ tsp. baking powder
- ¼ c. protein powder, chocolate, or vanilla flavor
- 2/3 c. unsweetened cocoa powder
- ¼ tsp. salt
- ½ c. unsalted butter, melted
- 4 large eggs
- ¾ c. heavy cream
- 1 tsp. vanilla extract

Nutritions: Calories: 253, Carbohydrates: 5.1g, Protein: 17.3g, Fat: 29.5g

120. Keto Crockpot Chocolate Lava Cake

Preparation:
30 Minutes

Cooking:
3 Hours

Servings:
12

Ingredients

- 1 ½ c. stevia sweetener, divided
- ½ c. almond flour
- 5 tbsps. unsweetened cocoa powder
- ½ tsp. salt
- 1 tsp. baking powder
- 3 whole eggs
- 3 egg yolks
- ½ c. butter, melted
- 1 tsp. vanilla extract
- 2 c. hot water
- 4 ounces sugar-free chocolate chips

Directions

1. Grease the inside of the Crock-Pot.
2. In a bowl, mix the stevia sweetener, almond flour, cocoa powder, salt, and baking powder.
3. In another bowl, mix the eggs, egg yolks, butter, and vanilla extract. Pour in the hot water.
4. Pour the wet ingredients into the dry ingredients and fold to create a batter.
5. Add the chocolate chips last.
6. Pour into the greased Crockpot and cook on low for 3 hours.
7. Allow to cool before serving.

Nutritions: Calories: 157, Carbohydrates: 5.5g, Protein: 10.6g, Fat: 13g

CHAPTER 17:
Tips on How to Live the Mediterranean Diet Lifestyle

We are all involved in being lean, losing weight, getting a good diet plan, and getting rid of cardiovascular and health-related illnesses. Typically, once you have a good diet plan such as the Mediterranean diet plan, the chances are that you will eventually reduce the number of calories in your body resulting in decreased heart-related issues.

The other benefits include weight shedding, fat burning and gradually slimming down. It is truly easy to implement diet plans like the Mediterranean diet plan. That's because you can't eat the gunk and bland vegetables that many people have to submit to just because they want to live longer and healthier.

You will enjoy delicious meals with the Mediterranean diet plan while still lowering the chances of getting heart-related problems. Here are a few tips to help adopt the Mediterranean diet.

1. Decide on a Diet Type

Most people tend to worry about their diet plans constantly. They worry if it will work, if they will lose weight, if they can reduce their chances of dying younger as a result of heart disease and cancer and, most importantly, worry if they can keep up with their diets. Okay, the thing is, if you really want to do this, you have to choose which choice you think works best for you.

There are two main dietary forms or regimens. You can do the planned kindor theDIY kind. It all depends on the makeup you have. For instance, some people don't like strict timetables and are more likely to fail to use them because they are instinctively opposed to things that make them feel like they're boxed in.

However, other people find it exciting to chart a strategy and are more likely to stick to it. It all depends on the person that you are. So, whatever happens, just pick one out. If you don't know which group you belong to, just go for one. You can always turn to the other if you don't like it.

2. Find Recipes That Will Work for You

Everybody's taste in food is different. You need to find and stick to that which works for you. The basic components of the Mediterranean diet plan include, among others, olive oil, legumes, vegetables, nuts, grains, unprocessed carbohydrates, fish, reduced red meat consumption, and saturated

fat.

Now, if you just like eating them like that, then it's all right. But if you want to make it much more fun, you'd have to find recipes that work. The South Beach Diet recipes, for example, are great and fun to cook. So, find recipes that inculcate these and which are based on the Mediterranean diet.

3. Get Creative with the Diet

After following a few diet plans, the reason many people return to eating junk is that the diets are either dull, repetitive, or lacking in flavor. So, what you should do is just go for those delicious meals. Get creative with the recipes. Try something new, and something different. Chances are if you're looking hard enough, you'll find lots of Mediterranean diet recipes that will last you for a whole year and more.

4. Be Disciplined

The Mediterranean diet is really simple to use and apply, so some would say it's hardly even a diet. I just see it as an alternative lifestyle that includes food choices that help you stay healthy and live longer. The secret, then, is discipline. Stay focused and who knows, you could just give yourself an extra 15 years of life and good health.

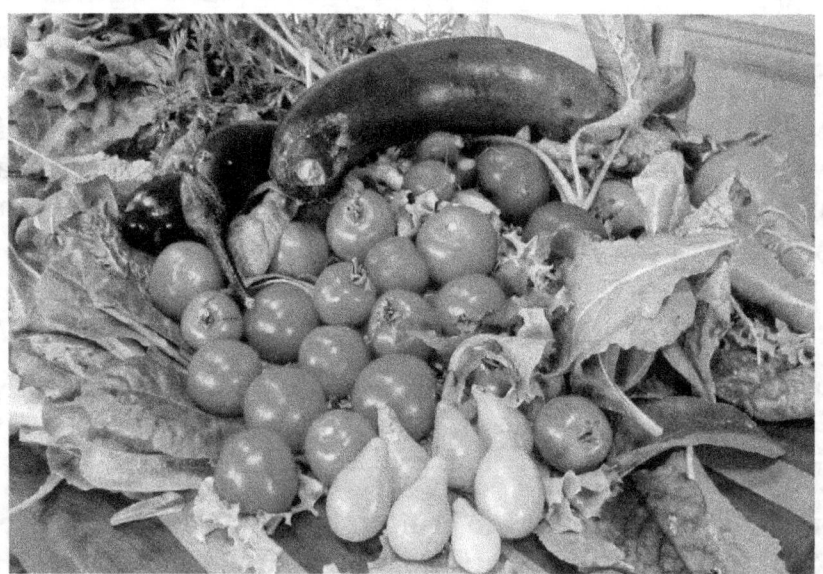

CHAPTER 18:
2-Week Meal Plan

Day	Breakfast	Lunch	Dinner	Dessert
1	Morning Oats	Mediterranean Cod Stew	Chicken Bolognese	Creamy Rice Pudding
2	Spinach Frittata	Herb Roasted Pork	Zoodles with Beet Pesto	Almond Cookies
3	Vanilla Pancakes	Caprese Chicken Dinner	Orange Fish Meal	Date and Nut Balls
4	Savory Egg Galettes	Kale Olive Tuna	Beef Tartare	Mango Snow
5	Artichoke Omelet	Vegetarian Coconut Curry	Simple Braised Pork	Watermelon Cream
6	Breakfast Toast	Mediterranean Beef Dish	Salmon Skillet Supper	Mascarpone and Fig Crostini

7	Bell Pepper Frittata	Meatballs and Sauce	Chicken Parm	Baklava and Honey
8	Vanilla Pancakes	Chicken Bolognese	Mediterranean Cod Stew	Almond Cookies
9	Artichoke Omelet	Chicken Parm	Kale Olive Tuna	Mango Snow
10	Savory Egg Galettes	Simple Braised Pork	Vegetarian Coconut Curry	Date and Nut Balls
11	Breakfast Toast	Beef Tartare	Caprese Chicken Dinner	Creamy Rice Pudding
12	Morning Oats	Meatballs and Sauce	Zoodles with Beet Pesto	Baklava and Honey
13	Spinach Frittata	Mediterranean Beef Dish	Orange Fish Meal	Mascarpone and Fig Crostini
14	Bell Pepper Frittata	Chicken Parm	Herb Roasted Pork	Watermelon Cream

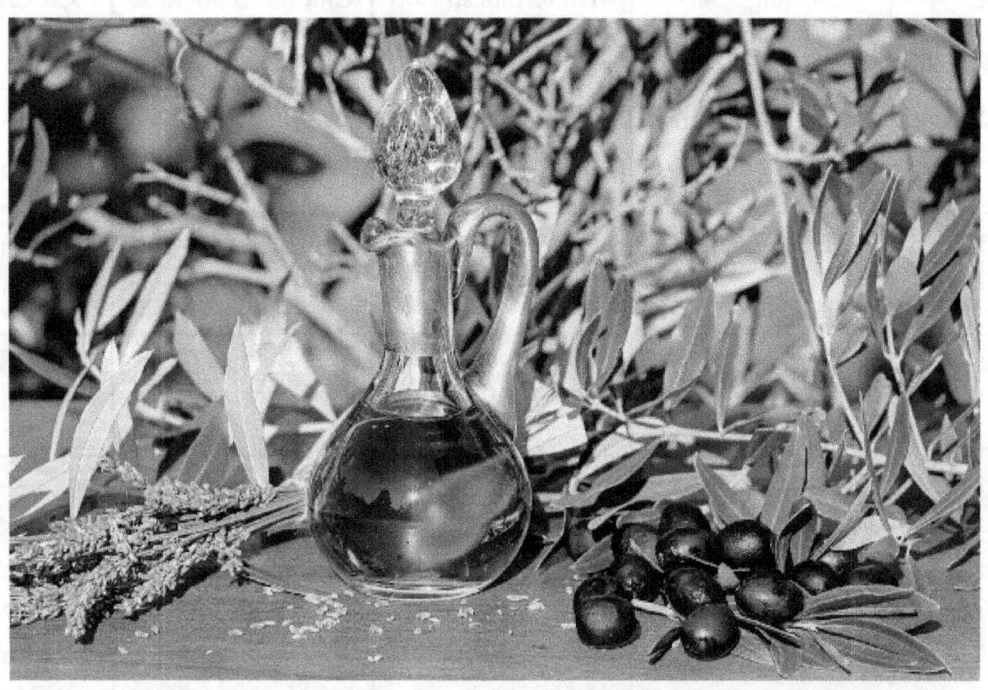

CONCLUSION

With the Mediterranean diet pattern, you will come closer to nature as the entire food concept depends on fresh produce. Mealtime, in these lands, is nothing short of a celebration. People living in these parts have a tradition of eating together. It is time to nurture interpersonal relations as well.

It is the right time to get into stride and do something that will improve your current state and give you a healthy future. After all, there is no more significant wealth than the health of an individual.

The goal was to provide a thorough look at this diet and all the advantages and disadvantages it can bring to your life. As always, when making dietary changes, you should consult your physician first to ensure this is a healthy change for you to achieve your goals regarding your health. With the Mediterranean diet, much research has proven it is the most efficient method to lose weight and improve your overall health.

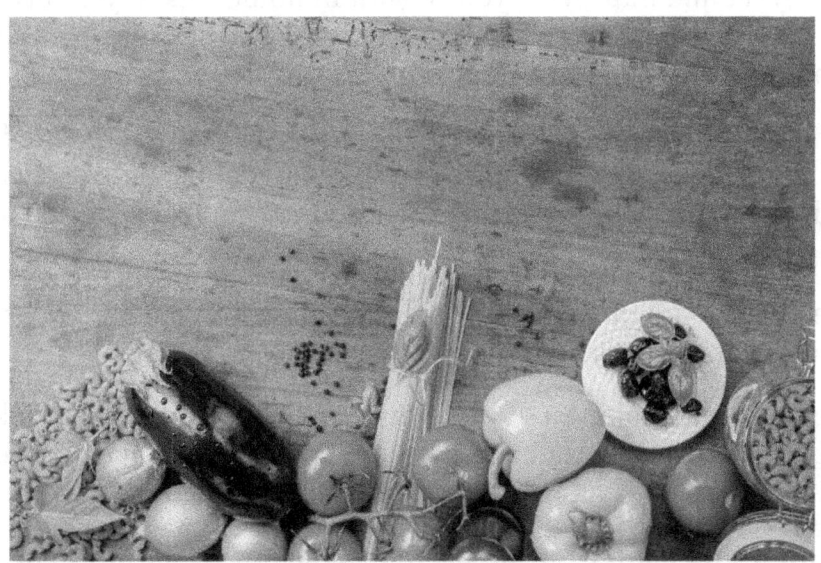

The primary aim of the Mediterranean diet is to make a person fit from within. Eating these foods will help enhance the outer physical appearance and bring out a healthy inner glow. People with cardiovascular issues, blood pressure, blood sugar, stress and anxiety, and stomach related ailments will benefit from this dietary program.

This cookbook will provide you with a detailed look at the Mediterranean lifestyle and exactly what it entails. The more informed you are about this diet and exactly what you should and should not be eating, the greater your chances of success will be!

Dishes that have a low quantity of meat are a significant part of the Mediterranean diet. It is customary among people from this region to include fresh fruit at the end of the meal. Cookies and cakes are not usually eaten daily. They are saved for some special celebrations and family gatherings. To keep your diet's emphasis more on the low quantity of saturated fat, replace the butter in your cakes, pastries, and cookies with olive oil wherever possible. Keep in mind, diversity and balance are the hallmarks of the Mediterranean diet, so serve dishes with a variety of tastes, temperatures, and textures. Numerous dishes taste best both ways, i.e., warm and cold. It prepares you for getting rid of the pressure to prepare a hot meal to serve. The recipes given in this book will make your work easy. It offers you an easy way to match your recipes.

All these Mediterranean dishes are worth trying. Some dishes are quick to make, but some will take time. When you have the final dish on your table, you will be satisfied with all the effort you put in. Do not hesitate to customize a little bit as per your preferences and health goals. People have been becoming more health-conscious nowadays, which is a pretty impressive thing to see in the modern world. To have a healthy lifestyle and to attain your goal of losing weight, the Mediterranean diet has become one of the most practiced fitness trends globally. Its popularity has increased with time. The Mediterranean diet is famously called a diet plan or a specific eating pattern. Research has shown that the Mediterranean diet can be one of the most potent tools for losing weight. It can effectively support you in fighting your belly fat and improving your health in numerous ways. Various studies have claimed that it improves brain health and decreases the risk of diabetes, cancer, and heart diseases. It can even help you to live a long and healthy life.

As long as you have this cookbook and stick to the simple rules of the Mediterranean diet, you can attain all the benefits it offers. One of the essential benefits of this diet is that it is perfectly sustainable in the long run, not to mention it is mouth-watering and delicious.

Once you start implementing this diet's various protocols, you will see a positive change in your overall health. Ensure that you are being patient with yourself and stick to your diet without making any excuses.

Shifting to a new diet and making a lifestyle change can be tough! This cookbook will allow you to gradually manage this journey and help you understand everything you need to know in this culinary tradition and finally benefit from it in the long run.

The Mediterranean diet allows you to get the chance to relish different kinds of meals.

There may be an emphasis on some particular food group, but none are excepted. Besides, this diet also allows you to have opportunities to know and cook more seasonal and fresh meals that will totally change your habits. Shifting to this lifestyle will give you a strong support system that you can rely on for years to come.

www.ingramcontent.com/pod-product-compliance
Lightning Source LLC
Chambersburg PA
CBHW081349080526
44588CB00016B/2423